WISDOM

A Manual for Nemonik Thinking

Dr Auke Schade

COPYRIGHT

First Edition
Published 25 April 2022
Dunedin, New Zealand
@ nemonik-thinking.org
ISBN 978-0-473-63078-2

FOREWORD

Technology has changed the static reality of the past into the hyperdynamic reality we live in today. Unfortunately, educational thinking did not adjust adequately to that revolution. Therefore, people have become static tinkers in a hyperdynamic reality. That systemic cognitive failure drives the Triangle of Doom. Education fosters science, science fosters technology, and technology fosters manmade extinction problems, such as nuclear war and climate change. That self-destruction is maintained by institutionalization, groupthink, and cognitive dissonance.

Nemonik Thinking (NT) is a unique paradigm of thinking that fosters new solutions for those old problems. NT is for the brain what Windows is for the computer. It is the first Cognitive Operating System (COS), because it tells the brain how-to-think, rather than what-to-think. The aim of NT is to maximize your success by applying Lao Zi's principle of dynamic balance. In his theory, success is to obtain what you seek and escape what you suffer [2] §62.

NT assigns the conscious to manage the mind and releases the subconscious genius by integrating rational, emotive, and intuitive thinking. It prepares, simplifies, defragments, and accelerates the memory and thinking processes with Dynamic Thinking and Mind Management.

Dynamic Thinking maximizes external success with an exhaustive checklist of 21 memorized prompts called nemoniks. They use guided-association to activate problem-solving tools such as: icons, definitions, synonyms, SWOT-analyses, questions, and proverbs relative to the particular situation.

Mind Management maximizes internal success with Concentrated-Relaxation and Mantras. Concentrated-Relaxation evokes semiconscious dominance. That mental state fosters the conscious management of the subconscious genius with mantras. A mantra is a short phrase that is silently repeated in the mind.

External success is measured within the physical reality of space, matter, and time. On the other hand, internal success is measured by the subjective perception of that external success. For example, the richest person could still feel poor, while the poorest one could feel rich. Hence, nemonik thinkers maximize both their external and internal success.

NT provides a competitive advantage for every human activity. It turns weaknesses into strengths and threats into opportunities by generating ideas, analyses, knowledge, and wisdom. It fosters a generation of nemonik thinkers focusing on success, balance, efficiency, and proactivity. They are always prepared. Therefore, they have higher panic-resistance and lower stress-levels. Nemonik Thinking might sound like magic, because it is [1].

I recommend you to upgrade to NT, because there is no valid and reliable alternative. Humanity is running out of time. Learn from my mistakes and start your training right now!

This manual provides you
with the wisdom
accumulated in proverbs.

CONTENTS

INTRODUCTION

This manual is about practical wisdom, rather than mystical philosophies. It is about the here and now. Nemonik Thinking aims to maximize success in your daily life by managing your mind with productive wisdom, logic, creativity, intuitions, skills, and emotions. In accord, Lao Zi defined success in his ancient *Dao De Jing* as: *"Obtain what you seek and escape what you suffer"* [1] §62. Therefore, mysticism and the supernatural are outside the scope of this manual.

Many heated arguments and conflicts are caused by using ambiguous concepts. In order to avoid such confusion about the wisdom for Nemonik Thinking, we have to define the key-concepts. First of all, there is a significant difference between knowledge and wisdom. Knowledge is a set of valid and reliable descriptions of reality. On the other hand, wisdom is the cognitive ability to apply that knowledge productively. Any fool could learn to split an atom, but only a wise person knows what to do with that knowledge.

Unfortunately, we live in an era in which sophisticated knowledge is applied without much wisdom. For example, manmade extinction problems, such as nuclear war and climate change, are the results of the counterproductive applications of knowledge. Fortunately, the accumulated wisdom of humanity is recorded in proverbs. Your ancestors paid for that wisdom with pain, blood, and tears. Only fools ignore their precious inheritance and keep reinventing the wheel. Therefore, that ancient wisdom is integrated and extended in Nemonik Thinking [2, 3].

Nemonik Thinking is unique mindware that aims to improve the working of the mind. Mindware is a set of rules, or algorithms, that tells the brainware how to create and maintain the mind. Mindware could be compared to the software of a computer. On the other hand, brainware is a set of material components comprising the Central Nerve System. Brainware could be compared to the hardware of a computer.

The mind is the nonmaterial part of a person that includes all conscious, semiconscious, and subconscious processes resulting from interactions between the brainware and mindware of that person. The conscious is the relatively small part of the mind that is dominant when awake; aware of the reality and the Self; and manages the mind. The semiconscious is the part of the mind that manages the communication between the conscious and subconscious. The subconscious is the largest part of the mind that is dominant when asleep; stores and processes bulk information; and is consciously inaccessible.

A computer operating system is the basic software that tells the electronic parts how to think as a computer. Similarly, a cognitive operating system is the basic mindware that tells the brain how to think, rather than what to think. Nemonik Thinking is the first true cognitive operating system. Nemonik Thinking is for your brain what Windows is for your computer.

Your external success is measured within the physical reality of space, matter, and time. On the other hand, your internal success is measured by your subjective perception of that external success. For example, the richest person could still feel poor, while the poorest one could feel rich. Hence, you have to maximize both your external and internal success. As shown in Figure 1: Nemonik Thinking is a cognitive tool that maximizes external success with Dynamic Thinking and internal success with Mind Management.

Figure 1: The structure of Nemonik Thinking.	
Nemonik Thinking *(maximize success)*	
Dynamic Thinking *(maximize external success)*	Mind Management *(maximize internal success)*

Dynamic Thinking is a cognitive tool that maximizes your external success by defragmenting your memory with a set of 21 nemoniks. A nemonik is a keyword that prompt the mind to recall associated information from memory and process that information in order to create new information.

Figure 2 shows the rationale for each of the 21 nemoniks. That set is exhaustive, because the nemoniks cover each aspect of thinking including: the cosmic principle, mind, reality, and the interaction between the mind and reality.

The nemoniks are like 21 library shelves that increase the efficiency of your memory by reorganizing the stored information by topic. In addition, Dynamic Thinking accelerates and improves your thinking with guided-association. Each consciously recalled nemonik activates automatically your subconscious in order to retrieve problem-solving tools including: the icon, definition, synonyms, SWOT-analysis, questions, and proverbs for that particular nemonik. Nevertheless, applying nemoniks without wisdom is counterproductive.

Figure 2: Hierarchy of Dynamic Thinking.

<table>
<tr><td rowspan="13">Dynamic Thinking</td><td>Phenomenon</td><td>Features</td><td>Nemoniks</td></tr>
<tr><td>Cosmos</td><td>Cosmic Principle (=)</td><td>Focus
Balance
Efficient
Proactive</td></tr>
<tr><td rowspan="2">Mind</td><td>Conscious</td><td>Objective
Collective</td></tr>
<tr><td>Subconscious</td><td>Creative
Reactive</td></tr>
<tr><td rowspan="3">Reality</td><td>Space</td><td>Advance
Stay
Retreat</td></tr>
<tr><td>Matter</td><td>Accumulate
Preserve
Dispose</td></tr>
<tr><td>Time</td><td>Act
Wait
Prepare</td></tr>
<tr><td rowspan="2">Interaction</td><td>Perception</td><td>Accept
Reject</td></tr>
<tr><td>Projection</td><td>Reveal
Conceal</td></tr>
<tr><td>Supernatural</td><td colspan="2">Outside the scope of DT</td></tr>
</table>

As shown in Figure 3: Mind Management is a cognitive tool that maximizes internal success with Concentrated-Relaxation and Mantras. Concentrated-Relaxation evokes semiconscious dominance. That mental state fosters the conscious management of the subconscious genius with mantras. A mantra is a short phrase that is silently repeated in the mind [2, 3].

Figure 3: Mind Management flowchart.

Conscious	◀affecters		**◀Subconscious**
▶	CR▶	**Semiconscious** dominance ▼	▲
▶	mantras▶	firewall▶	mindsets

CR = Concentrated-Relaxation

The aim of this manual is to provide a comprehensive set of proverbs for each of the 21 nemoniks. Studying and memorizing those proverbs will create guided-association between each nemonik and its associated wisdom. After sufficient study, consciously recalling a particular nemonik will provide automatically the memorized proverbs and their wisdom.

NEMONIK WISDOM

Focus

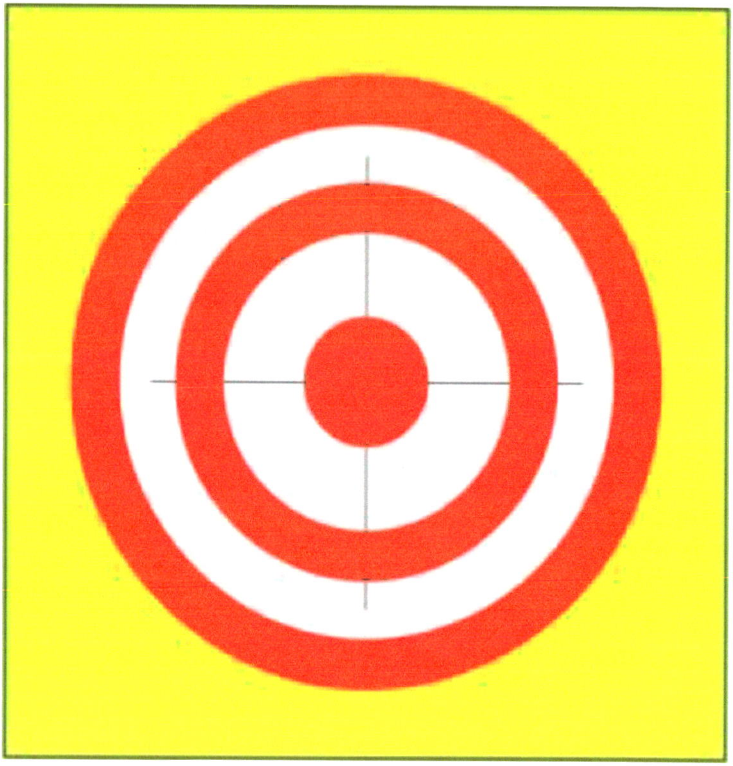

Mantra: I focus on success.

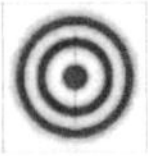

Description Focus

Focus is the nemonik that prompts your mind to ignore everything that could distract you from your goal.

Success is to obtain what you seek and escape what you suffer [1] §62. You can only maximize your success if you focus on your goals. Make sure that you know what to seek and what to avoid. Do not let other people replace your goals with their goals. The universe is fair: *If you ask for nothing then you will get nothing.*

Strength—focus concentrates all available resources on your goal.

Weakness—focus leaves no resources for alternatives and opportunities.

Opportunity—focus could maximize success despite the surrounding distractions.

Threat—focus could inhibit the consideration of valid alternatives (wearing blinkers). A strongly focused person could become a static thinker in a dynamic universe.

Wisdom relevant to Focus

A Jack of all trades is a master of none.

Before you can hit the target, you must select one.

Do not let others set your limits.

You reap what you sow.

Focus on obtaining what you seek
and escaping what you suffer [1] §62.

Circumstances alter cases.

Do not let others determine your limits.

Sages focus on past success,
rather than past failure.

Concentrate on things that work for you.

You cannot always get what you want.

Pursue the course that offers most advantages,
habit will soon make it agreeable and easy.

Do not focus so much on the lion
that you miss the snake.

Blessed are those who expect nothing,
because they will never be disappointed.

Focus on justice, rather than justifications.

Focus only on reason and you will lack compassion.

Concentrate on your goals, rather than obstacles.

Fame or life? What is closer?
Life or wealth? What is worth more?
Gain or loss? What hurts more [1] §44?

Do not live other people's dreams.

Fools have a good memory for bad things
and a bad memory for good things.

All roads lead to Rome.

Focus everything you got on your goal.

Turn weaknesses into strengths.

Focussed light burns through steel.

Success ruins a fool.

It is a weakness
if your focus blinds you
from seeing opportunities.

Failure is the mother of success.

Do not freeze your focus with dogmas.
The two hardest things in life to handle
are success and failure.

Enjoy your journey, but focus on your destiny.

Put your saddle on the right horse.

Focus on causes, rather than symptoms.

People and All-things concentrate on the Way.
It is the protection for competent people.
It is the sanctuary for incompetent people [1] §62.

Little things please little minds.

Focus your greatest strength on the weakest obstacle.

Success in life depends on how you handle your failures.

Concentrate on the present,
because the past is gone,
while the future has not arrived yet.

Apply consciously the twenty-one nemoniks
until they are a habit.

You are always correct;
whether you believe you can or you cannot.

Learn from yesterday, live today, focus on tomorrow.

Concentrate on substance, rather than its shadow.

Those who begin too many things finish none.

Concentrate on what is, rather than what should be.

A burden of one's own choice is never felt.

No good thing is a failure, and no evil thing is a success.

In handling their affairs,
people fail often close to their success.
Therefore, focus as careful
at the end as at the beginning.
Then affairs will not fail [1] §64.

If at first you do not succeed; try, try, and try again.

The fish will soon be caught that nibbles every bait.

Focus exclusively on obtaining what you seek
and you might not escape what you suffer.

The secret of success is constancy of focus.

You cannot be in two places at once.

No sage throws a spear without a target.

Concentrate on the changeable,
and accept the unchangeable.

What anyone has done; you can do.

A focus on beauty brings beauty during ugly times.

When you eat, focus on eating.
When you walk, focus on walking.

Obtaining what you seek is success,
but enjoying to obtain what you seek is happiness.

Better a big fish in a small pond,
than a small one in a big pond.

Focus exclusively on escaping what you suffer
and you might not obtain what you seek.

Do not desire the great splendour of jade,
but the grace of natural rock [1] §39.

The start of a journey
should never be mistaken for success.

Adjust your goal to the changing situation.

Do not let others set your goals.

Focus rejects distractions.

It is a poor goal
if it cannot be justified by success.

Follow your dreams and you prevent nightmares.

Question the question,
before you try to find an answer.

Need is the mother of industry.

One meets his destiny
often on the road taken to avoid it.

If destiny does not fit you,
fit yourself to destiny.

Be careful what you ask for,
because desire differs from possession.

Make your hobby your work,
and you will never work.

A goal that wins public praise is easier to reach.

If you cannot ride two horses at once,
then you should not be in the circus.

Focus on critical thinking,
rather than criticism.

You will live in the world you focus on.

Concentrate vital energy
and be as flexible as an infant [1] §10.

Responding to every thought spreads your focus thin.

Without a goal you might as well stay where you are.

In the dark, focus on the light.

The first step into the future is deciding what you want.

Eagles do not prey on small flies.

Better to be the head of a dog, than the tail of a lion.

Sages reject extremes,
reject grandeur,
and reject extravagance [1] §29.

Having a career is not the same as having a life.

Focus on the truth,
rather than winning arguments.

Turn threats into opportunities.

Use focus in combination with
balance, efficiency, and proactivity.

Do not sweat the small stuff.

Follow every impulse and you wander around in circles.

Eat to live, but do not live to eat.

Run after two hares and you will catch neither.

Focus on the wisdom of applying knowledge.

Take heed of the snake in the grass.

The road to hell is paved with good intentions.

Without wind, a vessel would not move.
Without a pilot, she would be lost.

Mistakes are stepping stones to success.

A focused thinker is never an average thinker.

Focus on your talents, and delegate the rest.

The universe is fair;
if you ask for nothing then you will get nothing.

Use rational thinking, rather than rationalizations.

Live not to eat, but eat to live.

Self-preservation is the first law of nature.

A clear goal is like a lighthouse.

What is worth doing is worth doing well.

The focus of a laser negates the inverse square law.

Do not put all your eggs in one basket.

Focus on hate and it will consume you.

Not even a sage can fulfil two missions at once.

Focus on solutions, rather than blame.

A person who runs after good fortune,
runs away from peace.

There is no success without focus.

Concentrate on removing extremes.
Nurture tranquillity diligently [1] §16.

If you sow wind, then you will reap the whirlwind.

Let the past take care of the past.

Concentrate all your mindpower on your goal.

A person who makes no mistakes makes nothing.

Just stop doing whatever is not working.

Success erases all the mistakes made along the way.

Enlarging the cake is more important than dividing it.

If you try to be in on everything, you will be in on nothing.

Constant dripping water wears away a stone.

The test of merit is success.

Fools hunt for misfortune.

Concentrate on the music and ignore the noise.

Use compassion, rather than detachment.

Aim higher than your target, because the arrow drops.

To focus on either happiness or sadness is your choice.

Between two stools you fall to the ground.

Do one new thing at the time.

The greatest achievement seems to be incomplete.
Yet, its usefulness is not reduced.
The greatest fullness seems to be empty.
Yet, its usefulness is never exhausted [1] §45.

Hang on tightly, and let go lightly.

Use dynamic thinking, rather than static thinking.

Sunrays do not burn until focused.

A focus without wisdom
is counterproductive..

Balance

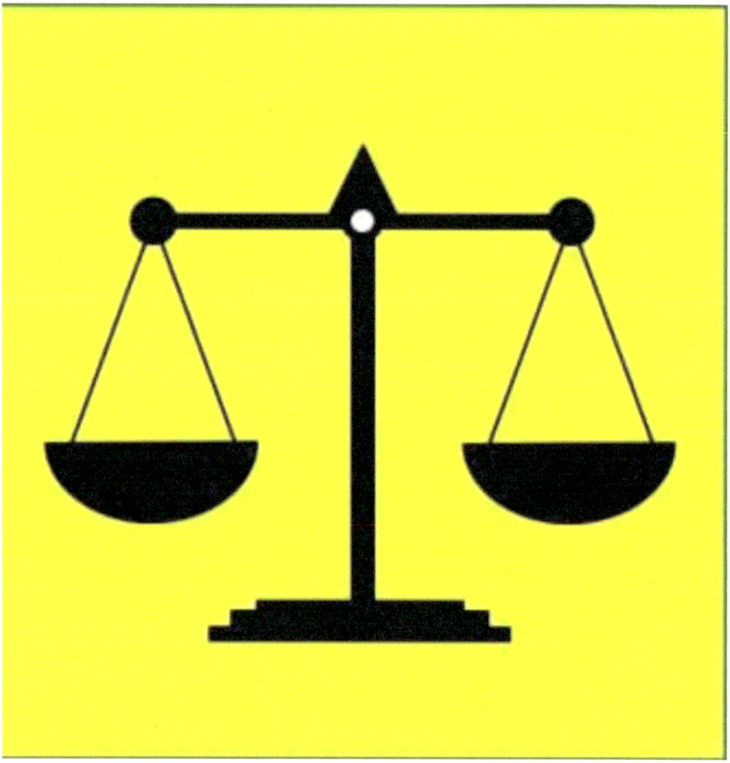

Mantra: I maintain the balance.

Description Balance

Balance is the nemonik that prompts your mind to maintain balance in order to avoid unproductive confrontations.

Any (Yin and Yang) difference creates vital energy (Qi) that restores their balance [1] §42. *Each action evokes a reaction of equal magnitude and opposite direction* [4]. Therefore, disturbing the balance is counterproductive. *Concentrate on removing extremes. Nurture tranquillity diligently* [1]§16. In modern terms: *Do not to rock the boat.*

Strength—maintaining the balance fosters productive mental and situational stability.

Weakness—maintaining the balance could maintain counterproductive mental and situational stability.

Opportunity—maintaining the balance could inhibit counterproductive reactions. *Any action evokes a reaction of equal strength and opposite direction* [4].

Threat—maintaining the balance could foster counterproductive apathy, procrastination, and complacency.

Wisdom relevant to Balance

Those who pelt others with pebbles
ask for stones in return.

Balance your desires and resources.

Prepare for the inevitable reaction
before you disturb the balance.

Matter and Antimatter
generate each other [1] §2.

Balance objectivity and creativity.

Enlightenment is the internal balance
between the conscious and subconscious.

Align with the forces of nature.
Align with the forces of people.

If you live by the sword,
then you die by the sword.

The end justifies the means.

Balance is the eternal principle of the universe.

Disturbing a balance
is like carrying water up the mountain.

The constancy of 'Nothingness'
maintains all Yin-Yang balances.

Balance objectivity and reactivity.

No rose without thorns.

Be humble for you are made of earth.
Be noble for you are made of stars.

Balance revealing and concealing.

Every cloud has a silver lining.

Work that disturbs the balance will be undone.

Create beauty and you create ugliness.

Chaos is the manifestation of restoring balance.

The equal sign (=) confirms
that balance is the principle of science.

Tranquillity is called returning to order.
Returning to order is a constant [1] §16.

Qi or Chi is the vital force
that balances Yin and Yang.

Rock the boat and you will get wet.

Live not only for yourself or only for others.

When things are the worst,
they begin to improve.

Moderation is the secret to lasting success.

Each action evokes an equal and opposite reaction.

Try to float and you sink; try to sink and you float.

Balance Yin and Yang.

No success without failure.

Wise men say only fools rush in.

Balance the weakness of age
with the strength of wisdom.

A heavy rock balanced on a needle
can be unbalanced by a butterfly.

Revenge evokes revenge.

A person who does many bad deeds
can expect a big one in return.

There is always opportunity cost.

The greatest threats
are having too much and too little.

Restoring a balance,
will create other imbalances.

If people desire to take the world
and interfere with it,
I see that they have no alternative.
The world is a container of energy
that cannot be interfered with [1] §29.

No bird flies on one wing.

If the world possesses the Way,
then racehorses will be kept for their manure.
If the world is without the Way,
then warhorses will be bred in the suburbs [1] §46.

One hand washes the other.

No joy is without sorrow.

Finish no dinner thirsty or drunk.

Returning to the roots is called tranquillity.
Tranquillity is called returning to order [1] §16.

Sages are good to those who are good.
They are also good to those who are bad.
So they gain goodness [1] §49.

Water is gold in the desert,
but the drowning person curses it.

Match collective needs with individual ones.

Balance action, waiting, and preparation.

Balance risks and rewards.

If you blame others for your failures,
then you should also give them credit for your successes.

Know the pure and observe the disgrace
and be the valley of the world [1] §28.

No morality without immorality.

Maintain the balance with moderation.

Balance advancing, staying, and retreating.

Forgive in order to restore your inner balance.

Spilling blood will be spilling blood.

Time restores every balance.

During bad fortune hold on,
during good fortune hold in.

Take the rough with the smooth.

No happiness without sadness.

Balance creativity and reactivity.

Who accepts nothing, has nothing to return.

Know the white and observe the black
and be the example for the world [1] §28.

No garden is without weeds.

Balance accumulation, preservation, and disposal.

Play with fire and you get burned.

Balance work and play.

Each storm returns to a calm and vice versa.

The Way of Nature is like flexing a bow.
High things are lowered.
Low things are raised.
It takes from those who have plenty.
It gives to those who have not enough [1] §77.

Nature balances without favouritism.

Bread borrowed should be returned.

Maintain the Yin-Yang balances.

You cannot change Yang
without nature changing Yin and vice versa.

Avoid extremes,
because rebalancing forces will destroy them.

Nothing is more destructive than living extremely.

You win a few, you lose a few.

Entropy is the manifestation of the force Qi or Chi,
which restores the Yin-Yang balances.

Nature will correct manmade imbalances.

Balance urgent issues with important ones.

Those who have plenty
and give to those in the world who have not enough
are the only ones who possess the Way [1] §77.

The more things change, the more they stay the same.

The thin end of the wedge is a dangerous extreme.

All-things around us rise,
and I watch them return [1] §16.

Use tranquillity without disgrace
and the world will regulate itself [1] §37.

Balance positivism with realism.

No pleasure without pain.

There are two sides to every story.

A natural balance is a balance in motion.

It is the Way of Nature
to take from what is plenty
and give to what is not enough.
However, the Way of People is different.
They take from what is not enough
and give to what is plenty [1] §77.

Harmonize the head with the heart.

The female always uses tranquillity
to overcome the male [1] §61.

Take into account the surrounding
natural and manmade balances.

You can always find fortune in your misfortune.

Sages trust those who trust them.
They also trust those who do not trust them.
So they gain trustworthiness [1] §49.

Fight fire with fire.

All-things carry Yin on their back
and carry Yang in their arms.
Any difference creates vital energy
that restores their harmony [1] §42.

Balance yourself and the world will follow.

The biter gets bitten.

No light without darkness.

The last drop makes the cup run over.

Desperate diseases call for desperate cures.

Karma is the reaction to your actions,
which restores the balance.

There are no rich without poor.

The eternal natural principle to success is balance.

What goes around comes around.

Too much is as bad as too little.

What goes up must come down.

Each tide returns to an ebb,
while each ebb returns to a tide.

If Marquises and Kings would follow the Way,
then All-things would submit themselves.
People would not have to be ordered,
but they would balance themselves [1] §32.

What is worth receiving is worth returning.

There is no competence without incompetence.

Payback is a bitch.

In the hour of great success,
the seeds of destruction are sown.

Create light and you create shadow.

Nature abhors a vacuum.

One good turn deserves another.

People who live in glass houses
should not throw stones.

Moderation in all things.

Without calling, things come [1] §73.

Sailing too sharp will capsize your boat.

The darkest hour is just before dawn.

Balance objectivity and collectivity.

It is easier to disturb the balance than to restore it.

Balance is the eternal principle of the universe.

Where ignorance is bliss it is folly to be wise.

Never do evil in the hope that good may come from it.

That which I receive, that I return.

Use balance in combination with
focus, efficiency, and proactivity.

The strong protect the weak and,
in return, the weak serve the strong.

The equal sign (=) represents the eternal natural balance.

Do not throw the spear that will return against you.

Bloodshed will cause bloodshed.

No gain without pain.

There are no sages without fools.

I am tranquil
and the people will perfect themselves [1] §57.

The last straw breaks the camel's back.

Cut your clothes according to your cloth.

Balance words with actions.

Concentrate on removing extremes.
Nurture tranquillity diligently [1] §16.

No life without death.

Ultimately, each balance will be restored
by either people or nature.

Returning to order is a constant.
Knowing this constant is brilliant.
Ignoring this constant is arrogant.
Arrogance causes misfortune [1] §16.

Even a worm will turn.

Know the male and observe the female
and become the stream of the world [1] §28.

The flow of water shows
the balancing force Qi or Chi in action.

Water is the embodiment of balance.

Do not get mad, but get even.

Reality is a system of interacting dynamic balances.

Blend listening with speaking.

One funeral makes many.

Death will balance all debts.

If you cannot increase your income,
then decrease your expenses.

The leaves of every tree return to the root when they fall.

Tranquillity is the sovereign of rashness [1] §26.

Do not take a gun to kill a mosquito.

Desire is the core of manmade imbalances.

Balance accepting and rejecting.

Fortune gives and takes.

Inner balance is the foundation of self-confidence.

Maintaining the balance
without wisdom
is counterproductive.

Efficient

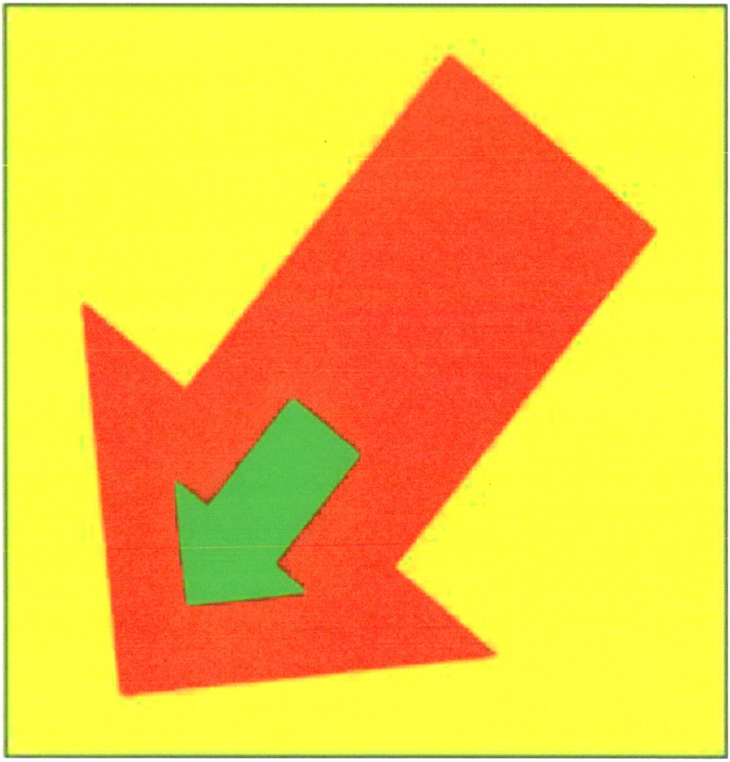

Mantra: I go with the flow.

Description Efficient

Efficiency is the nemonik that prompts your mind to achieve your goal with a minimum of resources.

When effort is needed, then there is never enough to take the world [1] §48. Effort is an indication of counterproductive inefficiency. *Therefore, sages manage their affairs with Efficiency* [1] §2. *Act with Efficiency. Work without effort* [1] §63. In modern terms: *Go with the flow.*

Strength—efficiency reduces the time, effort, and resources required to reach your goal.

Weakness—efficiency inhibits the focus on your goal if you *go with the flow.*

Opportunity—efficiency could help you to succeed in difficult situations. It could preserve resources for future problems.

Threat—efficiency could alienate you from other people. It can be inhumane, unkind, cold, controlling, bureaucratic, and robotic. Efficiency is doing things right, but it is not necessarily doing the right things.

Wisdom relevant to Efficient

Effort is a sign of inefficiency.

The beaten road is the safest.

Hammer it too sharp
and it cannot last long [1] §9.

Do not grasp things by the blade.

Make the best of a bad job.

Do not put the cart before the horse.

Bent like a reed to the storm.

Going with the raging river
will never bring you to the top of the mountain.

Speaking is silver, but listening is gold.

One nail drives out another.

A person who solves a problem with a problem;
will always have a problem waiting.

Do not keep more cats than will catch mice.

Another one's misfortune does not cure your pain.

Work smarter, rather than harder.

Better the devil you know, than the devil you do not.

Maximize your profit.

Fight fire with fire.

Sages pay attention to what matters most.

If one wants to take the world,
then one should always use no effort.
When effort is needed,
then there is never enough to take the world [1] §48.

Efficient production methods make workers obsolete.

Stretch your arm no further than your sleeve.

Stop doing what is not working.

Let the force (Qi) be with you.

Teaching without speaking and Non-action
will benefit the whole world [1] §43.

Drink down your sorrow and it returns the morning after.

Do not pour water into a basket
and expect it to remain there.

Attend to the big picture that maximizes your success.

Attend to details if that maximizes your success.

One cannot put back the clock.

Do not try to reinvent the wheel.

Nothing in the world is as soft and weak as water.
Yet, in attacking hard and strong things,
nothing has a greater ability to overcome them.
Therefore, nothing could replace its purpose [1] §78.

Humanity's efficiency is undone by population growth.

Cross the stream where it is shallowest.

Apply creative thinking to new problems.

Give a person a fish and he eats for a day.
Teach a person to fish and he eats for a lifetime.

You cannot get blood out of a stone.

Effective is doing the right thing,
while efficiency is doing the thing right.

Those who act will fail.
Those who hold will lose.
Therefore, sages will use Non-action [1] §64.

It is ill jesting with sharp swords.

Align with the force Qi.

Do not bark yourself if you have a dog.

The universe might help sailors in a storm,
but they must stay at the wheel.

Never trouble trouble, until trouble troubles you.

Fools do not accept reality.

The best is the enemy of the good.

The eye of the master does more work than his hands.

Act with a silent mind.

Nothing succeeds like success.

Cut diamond with diamond.

A bird in the hand is worth two in the bush.

Get the greatest good out the greatest evil.

Do not exhaust yourself by swimming upstream.

Let sleeping dogs lie.

Great people use little effort.

Act without great action.

Never do things by halves.

Apply objective thinking to the laws of nature.

Do not cut the branch you sit upon.

Apply the twenty-one nemoniks to each situation.

Do not make a stick to beat your own back.

Competent accountants
do not use bamboo counting sticks [1] §27.

Luck is besotted with the efficient.

It is ineffective
to complete counterproductive tasks efficiently.

When misfortune sleeps, let no one wake her.

Let well alone.

It is ill striving against the stream.

Do not buy a cow when the milk is cheap.

Competent wardens lock without keys.
Yet, it cannot be opened [1] §27.

Better to avoid missing, than hitting a hundred times.

Those who make rash promises
are certainly difficult to trust.
Those who regard everything as easy
will have certainly many difficulties.
Therefore, sages regard everything as difficult.
Hence, they have no difficulties in the end [1] §63.

Use the natural and artificial balances to your advantage.

If it is not broken, do not fix it.

Act with Non-action,
then there will be no anarchy [1] §3.

I use no effort
and the people will become
wealthy by themselves [1] §57.

Align with the rebalancing forces.

Of two evils, choose the lesser one.

Do not bite the hand that feeds you.

Minimize your losses.

Wake not a sleeping lion.

Superior virtue uses Non-action
and there is no action used [1] §38.

Easy does it.

Turn threats efficiently into opportunities.

Act with Non-action. Work without effort [1] §63.

There are no birds in last year's nest.

Do not repair what is not broken.

The world is a container of energy
that cannot be interfered with [1] §29.

Use no effort when taking the world [1] §57.

People have created efficient ways to kill each other.

Sages win the war before it starts.

To succeed, one must adjust to the situation.

Efficiency fosters mindless repetition.

Speed and accuracy do not agree.

The falconer feeds only the birds he needs.

Take things as you find them.

Efficiency preserves resources.

It takes a thief to catch a thief.

Sail your boat, rather than rowing it.

Do not use soldiers to force the world.
Such actions are likely to rebound [1] §30.

Balance efficiency with compassion.

Birds do not foul their own nest.

The best thing hurts when it is grabbed by the blade.

Solve a person's problem
and that person lives another day.
Teach that person to think
and that person becomes a survivor.

Flapping its fragile wings,
a butterfly could create an unstoppable tornado.

Turn weaknesses efficiently into strengths.

Do not push the river, it will flow by itself.

If the mind is not effective yet,
then fear that it will cease [1] §39.

The misfortune of a fool is a warning to the wise.

Increased efficiency increases the production,
while increased production increases the population.

Misfortunes should not to be awakened.

Trust your hidden genius.

Sages manage their affairs with Non-action [1] §2.

Change that what is not working.

A place for everything,
and everything in its place.

Show that you work hard,
and you show that you are not fit for the job.

You cannot make a silk purse out of a sow's ear.

Efficiency without effectiveness is counterproductive.

What cannot be cured must be endured.

Efficiency fosters inhumanity.

Do not start a fight that you cannot win.

Learn from the mistakes of others,
rather than from your own.

Do the right thing right.

Nothing is done, while something remains undone.

There is always someone better in something.

Apply collective thinking to the laws of people.

Go with the flow.

Sages select the right horse for the course.

Make a small ripple that creates a huge tsunami.

If you want a thing well done, then delegate it.

Apply reactive thinking to repetitive problems.

Perfection is measured in your ability to adjust.

A rising tide lifts all boats.

It is useless
to tell a river that it runs in the wrong direction;
just swim in the direction it runs.

When two dogs fight for a bone, a third runs away with it.

An eagle can soar, because it aligns with the rising air.

Use efficiency in combination with
focus, balance, and proactivity.

In the Vatican, it is inefficient to strive with the Pope.

Avoid overkill, because that will cause overreaction.

Laziness is the hallmark of efficiency.

If you have no time, then become more efficient.

Concentrate vital energy
and be as flexible as an infant [1] §10.

Do not just aim; but hit the target.

Do not meet trouble half way.

I practice Non-action
and the people will transform themselves [1] §57.

If a thing is worth doing, then it is worth doing well.

Minimize your time, efforts,
and resources to reach your goal.

The Way of Nature has no favourites.
It is always with the competent people [1] §79.

Do not try to make frozen water ripple.

Floating downstream is effortless.

Let the smith stick to his anvil.

A reed bending to the wind lives on, while mighty oaks fall.

What is done well is quick enough.

Change direction,
if that direction requires too much effort.

Efficiency without compassion is inhumane.

Be careful,
because each person
descends from a unbroken line of survivors.

Light a candle, rather than cursing the darkness.

Be aware that the flow you follow
might divert from your goal.

Efficiency without wisdom
is counterproductive.

Proactive

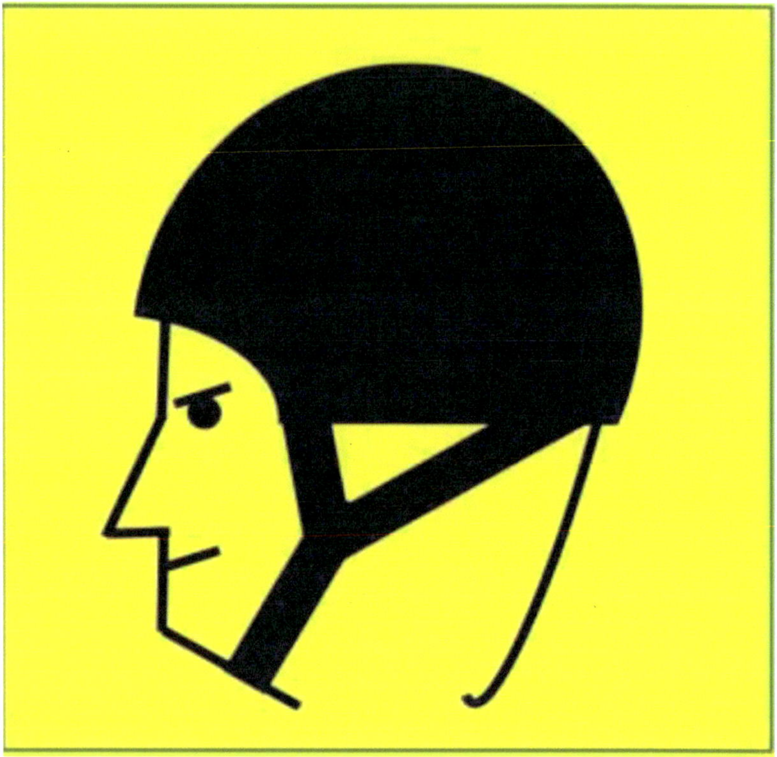

Mantra: I prevent.

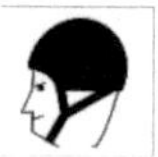

Description Proactive

Proactive is the nemonik that prompts your mind to act early in order to prevent the escalation of problems.

That what is at rest is easy to hold. That what is not manifest is easy to plan. That what is fragile is easy to break. That what is small is easy to scatter. Act when it has not happened yet. Control it when it is not chaotic yet. A tree that takes both arms to embrace grows from a little cutting [1] §64. In modern terms: *Prevention is the best cure.*

Strength—proactivity inhibits problems to grow out of control. *Prevent, rather than cure.*

Weakness—proactivity fosters a focus on all new problems that will reduce the focus on your specific goal.

Opportunity—proactivity could preserve your resources for unpredictable problems you might face in the future.

Threat—proactivity fosters rash actions that could backfire and destroy future opportunities. *Problems might be opportunities in disguise.* Correct timing is crucial for any action.

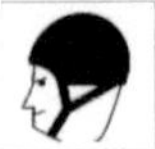

Wisdom relevant to Proactive

Tiny threats can have great consequences.

The weakness of proactivity
is the difficulty to predict the future.

Turn threats early into opportunities.

The sooner begun, the sooner done.

Good care prevents accidents.

Act when it has not happened yet.
Control it when it is not chaotic yet [1] §64.

Get up early so that you do not have to stay up late.

Seeds planted determine your harvest.

Better proactive at the beginning, than reactive at the end.

Setting the conditions
before you make an agreement
is better than having an argument
in the middle of the work.

Proaction is preventive action.

Ill weeds grow quickly.

Better to prevent than regret.

Sages do now, what fools do later.

When you want rice, you have to plant rice.

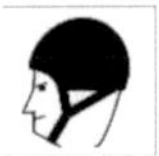

A tree that takes both arms to embrace
grows from a little cutting.
Nine-tenth of a tower
rises from a simple basket of earth.
A thousand meters height
starts from under your feet [1] §64.

Nurture opportunities when they are still small.

A stitch in time saves nine.

Predict the rebalancing forces and you predict the future.

Pursue the difficult, while it is easy.
Act large, while it is still small.
The world's most difficult things arise from the easiest.
The world's largest things arise from the smallest.
Therefore, all sages will avoid great actions.
Hence, they can achieve greatness [1] §63.

Lock the stable-door before the horse is gone.

Great oaks grow from little acorns.

Create space for things to happen.

Use all nemoniks early
to analyse the situation of all stakeholders.

The beginning determines the end.

One does not instruct a child on return;
one instructs a child when going.

Do the best now in order to be the best tomorrow.

A small threat requires only a small action.

Turn weaknesses early into strengths.

A neglected duty returns tomorrow
with seven others on its back.

Prevent blame and guilt with timely action.

Do not wait for an anthill to become a mountain.

Prevention is the best cure.

Procrastination kills proactivity.

Weak people wait for opportunities,
strong people create them.

A huge building starts with one bucket of earth.

Act like you are what you want to be.

Each proaction will evoke an equal and opposite reaction.

Do today in order to survive tomorrow.

Do not grow weeds that cover your dreams.

Your future depends on your actions right now.

Preventing to get stuck is proactive.

That what is at rest is easy to hold.
That what is not manifest is easy to plan.
That what is fragile is easy to break.
That what is small is easy to scatter [1] §64.

The longest journey starts with one step.

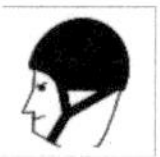

Proactivity reduces anxiety.

Rhinoceroses have no place to ram their horns.
Tigers have no place to strike their claws.
Soldiers have no place to thrust their swords.
What is the reason?
Because sages avoid the realm of death [1] §50.

It is easier to prevent ill habits than to break them.

An ounce of prevention is worth a pound of cure.

Sages set their destiny before they start running.

Paranoia poisons proactivity.

Aim before you shoot.

It is better to prevent than having a great remedy.

If we knew where death resided,
we would never stay there.

Get an umbrella before it rains.

Even an optimist should wear a helmet during a war.

Plan your action in advance.

Balance proactivity with patience.

Each tsunami starts with a small ripple.

The hand that rocks the cradle rules the world.

It is better preventing than fixing.

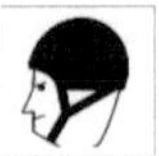

A good start is half the work.

Avoid, rather than avenge.

Good watch prevents misfortune.

Opportunity seldom knocks twice.

Superior generals position themselves,
rather than fight (Sun Zi).

The best doctor prevents illness,
an average doctor visits when the illness is imminent,
and the unskilled doctor treats your illness.

Use proactivity in combination with
focus, balance, and efficiency.

If you do not grow food then you will not eat.

Today's action prevents tomorrow's disaster.

Preventing people from falling is better
than helping them to get up.

Use all nemoniks early to analyse your situation.

Do not wait to be chosen, but choose yourself.

Prepare, rather than repair.

Those who pretend to know the future
are the fruitless flowers of the Way
and the chiefs of fools [1] §38.

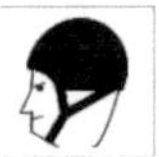

The early bird catches the worm.

Remove the stone and you won't stumble.

Proactivity without wisdom
is counterproductive.

Objective

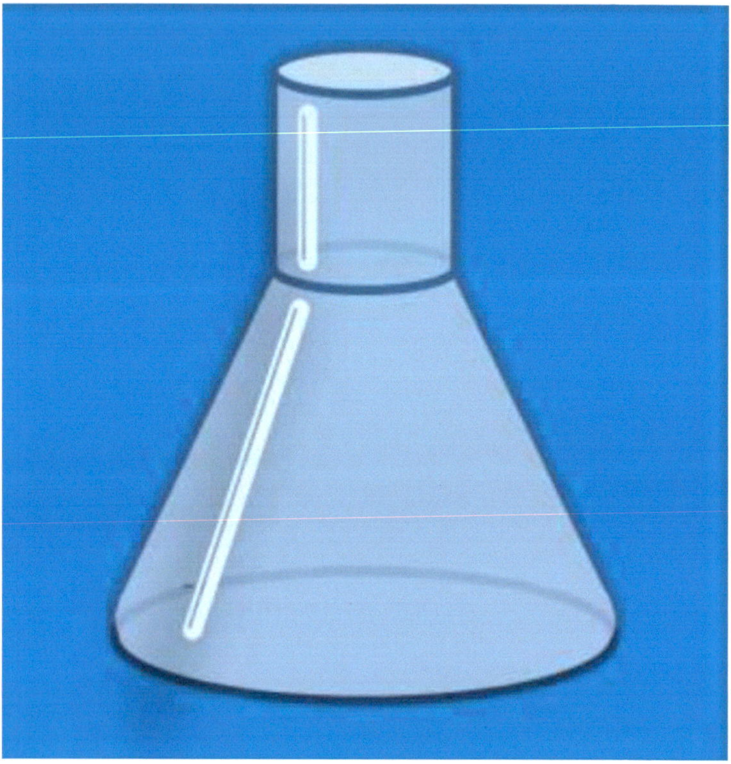

Mantra: I align with nature.

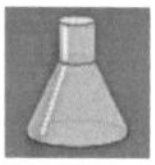

Description Objective

Objective is the nemonik that prompts your mind to deal with the natural part of reality.

The Way of Nature has no favourites. It is always with the competent people [1] §79. Lao Zi's Way of Nature refers to the objective laws of modern physics. Objective is a description of reality that is independent of what anyone believes. The objective mindmode uses conscious rational thinking in order to turn the immutable laws of nature into science.

Strength—objective thinking reveals the laws of nature, which fosters predictions.

Weakness—objective thinking is a journey, rather than a destiny. Therefore, the objective truth is temporal, rather than eternal.

Opportunity—objective thinking could foster survival through scientific development.

Threat—objective thinking could foster manmade extinction problems. Rationalizing conclusions could replace rational thinking. Criticizing others could replace critical thinking. Peer reviews could become peer pressure fostering groupthink.

Wisdom relevant to Objective

Science is the child of reason and logic.

Eternal truth is the prime measure.

Absence of evidence is no evidence of absence.

Wisdom is the productive application of knowledge.

No one has to believe in logic, because it is self-evident.

Nature does not punish or reward,
it presents consequences.

It is hard to be objective to the end.

A short defenition prevents a long debate.

Self-doubt is the beginning of objectivity.

If all alternative explanations are eliminated,
then the truth remains.

A short definition prevents a long debate.

Facts are illusions built on assumptions.

Let the people always be without knowledge
and without desire [1] §3.

Knowledge is power,
but knowledge without wisdom is madness.

Test whether repetition provides the same result.

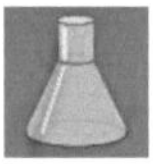

Replacing objectivity with authority leads to disaster.

Sages do not travel and yet they know.
They do not see and yet they name.
They do not act and yet they achieve [1] §47.

Foster the wisdom to know
the difference between the possible and impossible.

Use your objective mindmode
in combination with your
collective, creative, and reactive mindmodes.

Discard adoration and reject knowledge
and the people will benefit a hundred times [1] §19.

Make sure that your facts are valid and reliable.

Empirical research without a theory
is as a ship without a rudder.

We must convince with reason, not enforce with dogmas.

Those who know do not speak.
Those who speak do not know [1] §56.

Know the male and observe the female
and become the stream of the world [1] §28.

Science is truth in motion.

The strength of science is objective facts,
while the weakness of science is
the subjective interpretation of those facts.

A little knowledge is a dangerous thing.

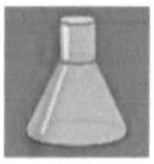

Wisdom is
the productive application
of knowledge.
Enlightenment is the balance
between the conscious (yang)
and the subconscious (yin).
One who is not enlightened
cannot be wise.

Focus on facts, rather than rhetoric.

When you rely too much on reason,
you end up not relying enough on feeling.

Fools try to adjust the objective reality
to their subjective beliefs.

Science is not a democracy.

Garbage in garbage out.

Know the pure and observe the disgrace
and be the valley of the world [1] §28.

An educated guess is only a subjective opinion.

Objectivity requires freedom of thinking.

Common sense is not that common.

Do not leave home
in order to learn about the world.
Do not look through the window
in order to learn about the Way of Nature [1] §47.

Keep it simple stupid!

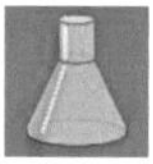

People are difficult to rule
if they use their knowledge [1] §65.

The development of science fosters inevitably the
specialization that destroyed Babel.

Sages adjust their subjective beliefs
to the objective reality.

Test whether the applied if-then-statements
are valid and reliable.

Truth is stranger than fiction.

Logic is the only way to challenge belief-systems.

Understand the surroundings without
using knowledge [1] §10.

Groupthink inhibits the objective mindmode.

Logical evidence inhibits false beliefs.

Custom without reason is only an ancient mistake.

Using knowledge to rule the country
is betraying the country.
Using no knowledge to rule the country
is benefiting the country [1] §65.

Fools reject logical arguments by rejecting logic.

Sages do not desire
to display their knowledge [1] §77.

Science is based on probabilitics,
rather than objective facts.

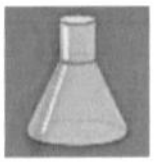

Science cannot prove that a phenomenon does not exist.

Everything happens for a reason.

Logical arguments comprise a set of objective facts
leading to an irrefutable conclusion.

Find the truth by experimentation.

A fact is a description of reality,
which is supported by sensory perception or logic.

Those who daily pursue knowledge will expand.
Those who daily pursue the Way will contract.
Contract and contract until there is Non-action left.
There is no action and yet there is action [1] §48.

Objectivity refers to the past, rather than the future.

Do not value knowledge
and the people will not strive [1] §3.

Love the people and rule the country
without using knowledge [1] §10.

Test whether the conclusion is valid and reliable.

Find the truth with repetition.

Use logic to solve natural problems.
Use compassion to solve artificial problems.

The Way of Nature has no favourites.
It is always with the competent people [1] §79.

Those who know are not educated.
Those who are educated do not know [1] §81.

Reason succeeds where force fails.

Repetition shows the objective truth.

Knowing that you do not know earns respect.
Not knowing that you do not know is a weakness.
Therefore, sages are not weak.
They consider their weakness as a weakness.
Hence, it is not a weakness [1] §71.

Logic and passion do not travel together.

The more people know,
the stranger the things they begin to develop [1] §57.

Objectivity is independent of anyone's belief.

Reason is the language of objective thinking.
Rhetoric is the language of collective thinking.

Discard knowledge and there are no worries [1] §19.

In the country of the blind, the one-eyed person is king.

Cognitive dissonance inhibits the objective mindmode.

Claiming objectivity
without logical evidence is false rhetoric.

Let those who know, not dare to act but stop [1] §3.

Find the truth by observation.

Logic challenges beliefs with irrefutable evidence.

There is no logic without objective facts.

Without common sense, there is no room for good advice.

Your objective mindmode cannot function
without objective facts.

Fools argue that their opinions are facts,
while the facts of others are opinions.

Know the white and observe the black
and be the example for the world [1] §28.

Science is not a democracy with voting rights,
therefore, consensus does not count.

The proof is in eating the pudding.

Those who know other people are wise.
Those who know themselves are brilliant [1] §33.

Knowing harmony is called the constant.
Knowing the constant is called brilliance [1] §55.

Apply your objective mindmode to the laws of nature.

A person without reason is a beast in season.

There is nothing new under the sun.

Check whether all alternatives are eliminated.

Who does not listen to reason cannot apply reason.

Facts are stubborn.

The objective mindmode is conscious and rational.

Objectivity has no room for miracles.

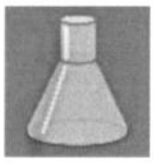

Check whether the 'and-, or- and nor-statements'
are valid and reliable.

Eliminate fiction until the truth remains.

The more that people travel far away the less they know.
Therefore, sages do not travel and yet they know.
They do not see and yet they name.
They do not act and yet they achieve [1] §47.

Sages know themselves,
but do not display themselves [1] §72.

Science is a journey, rather than a location.

Check your fact, before you act.

Test whether the supporting statements of the argument
are valid and reliable.

A true argument is consistent, valid, and reliable.

**Objectivity without wisdom
is counterproductive.**

Collective

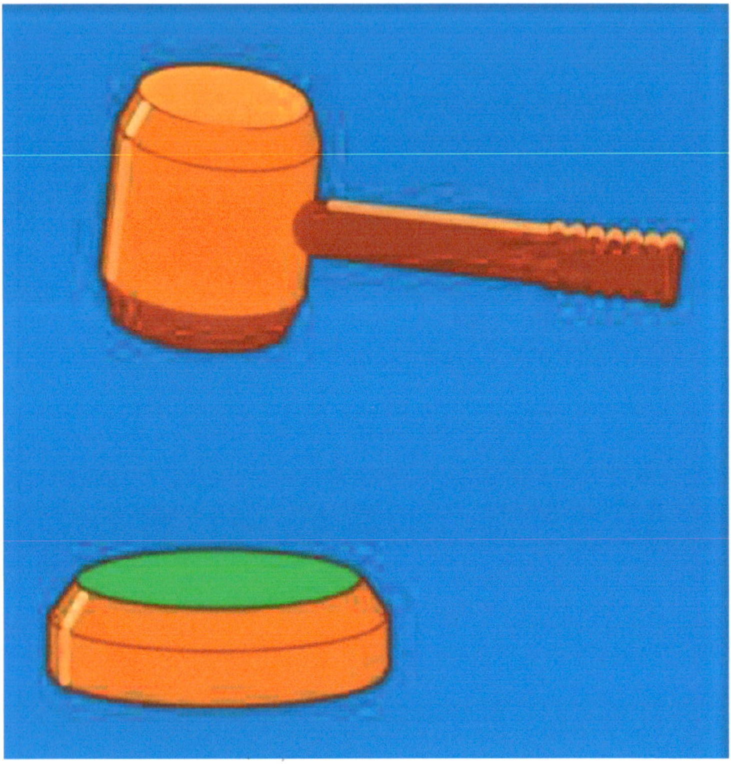

Mantra: I unite with people.

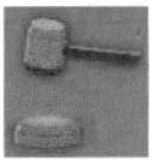

Description Collective

Collective is the nemonik that prompts your mind to deal with the artificial or manmade part of reality.

When people do not fear authority, then greater authority will appear [1] §72. A collective is an organized group of people with a common goal such as a family, business, tribe, nation, society, or the entire human race. The collective mindmode uses conscious rational thinking in order to create the law and order that formalizes human interaction.

Strength—collective thinking creates human law and order, which fosters the prediction of people's behaviour.

Weakness—collective thinking fosters enforcement of the law, dissidence, and rebellion.

Opportunity—collective thinking could foster a productive cooperation within the collective.

Threat—collective thinking could foster strict rules that cause collective stagnation in a dynamic universe. In order to control dissidents, the rules could become inhumane, unkind, cold, controlling, and bureaucratic.

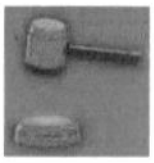

Wisdom relevant to Collective

The collective is the child of law and order.

Innocent until proven guilty.

Reasonable doubt is the prime measure.

Honour your father and your mother.

Do not steal.

Do not murder.

Do not commit adultery.

Do not foster false withness.

Do not seek what belongs to others.

Before claiming respect, give respect.

Before claiming rights, fulfill your obligations.

Nature does not recognize any collective rights.

The price for collective protection
is the loss of personal freedom.

Possession is nine-tenth of the law.

Friends should feel free to scold and give advice.

It needs more skill than I can tell,
to play the second fiddle well.

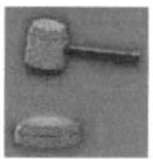

A stream cannot rise above its source.

Do not dare to take power [1] §30.

If you have a good friend, then you do not need a mirror.

A divided house cannot stand.

Rights cannot be claimed,
because any right has to be given by someone else.

Leave the door open for reconciliation.

Accept the country's shame
and be called the Kingdom's leader.
Accept the country's misfortune
and be called the world's King [1] §78.

Familiarity breeds contempt.

No agreement is reached
when it is reached under pressure.

If Marquises and Kings do not use superior nobility,
then fear that they will be overthrown [1] §39.

United we stand, divided we fall.

Reward productive behaviour.

When the blind lead the blind,
both shall fall into the ditch.

Before claiming respect, act with respect.

Everybody's business is nobody's business.

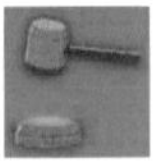

Do not bring grief to yourself by giving pleasure to others.

When the Emperor is crowned
and the three ministers are installed,
a millstone of jade preceded by four horses,
is not as good as sitting down
and presenting this [1] §62.

The collective mindmode is conscious and semi-rational.

A willing helper does not wait until he is asked.

Set a beggar on horseback and he will ride to the devil.

Right carried too far becomes wrong.

Before claiming leadership
know where to go.

Where there is negotiation,
there is hope for agreement.

If people always fear certain death,
then there is always someone in charge
of executing them [1] §74.

If you share other people's wealth,
try to lessen their misfortune.

A dogma is a collective statement
that cannot be challenged by an individual.

Every person has a price.

When people do not fear authority,
then greater authority will appear [1] §72.

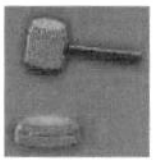

The dancers must pay the fiddler.

Be tranquil
and the people will perfect themselves [1] §57.

Do not ask for a favour
when someone else has just been rejected one.

You can close the city gates,
but you cannot close the people's mouths.

Let the people always be
without knowledge and without desire [1] §3.

Human law should treat all monks the same way.

You cannot run with the hare and hunt with the hounds.

Never reward counterproductive behaviour.

Little thieves are hanged by the great ones.

People take death lightly,
because they seek to live substantially.
Therefore, they take death lightly.
Only those who do not act for the purpose of living
are knowledgeable at valuing life [1] §75.

New lords, new laws.

Some might take the lower position
to associate.
Others might be in the lower position
to associate [1] §61.

Desire not to desire and the people
will become simple by themselves [1] §57.

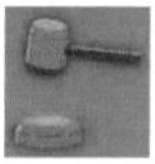

Many are called, but few are chosen.

People prefer the narrow winding roads.
Their palaces are very clean.
Their fields are overgrown with weeds.
Their storehouses are very empty [1] §53.

Use justice when ruling the State.
Use surprise when employing armies.
Use no effort when taking the world [1] §57.

Kings have long arms.

Give fools an inch and they will try to take a yard.

When in Rome do as the Romans.

Replacing objectivity with authority leads to disaster.

Only those who do not strive
will therefore not fail [1] §8.

Competent people
are the teachers of incompetent people.
Incompetent people
are the resources of competent people [1] §27.

One cannot demand rights without accepting obligations.

If they are not with you, then they are against you.

Rhetoric succeeds where force fails.

The cost of law inhibits justice.

Rhetoric is the language of collective thinking.
Logic is the language of objective thinking.

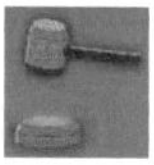

Jack is as good as his master.

Injustice justifies rebellion.

What everybody fears, one has to fear as well [1] §20.

Justice is hard to define, while injustice is obvious.

Birds in their little nest agree.

The first duty of a soldier is obedience.

If people would sweep their own doorstep
then the city would be clean.

Union is strength.

Human law is only as good as its gatekeepers.

Anyone makes a good enemy,
but not everyone makes a good ally.

Human law without enforcement is counterproductive.

Forced kindness deserves no thanks.

The sharp weapons of the State
should not be used in view of the people [1] §36.

You cannot please everyone.

The high must use the low as their foundation [1] §39.

It is better to reward productive behaviour,
than to punish counterproductive behaviour.

Without laws; people are animals and the criminal is King.

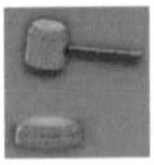

Four eyes see more than two.

It is the Way of Nature
to take from what is plenty
and give to what is not enough.
However, the Way of People is different.
They take from what is not enough
and give to what is plenty [1] §77.

The law is a negotiable agreement
between members of the collective.

Do-gooders do only good in order to gain collective praise.

When the flag is unfurled,
then all reason is in the trumpet.

Necessity knows no law.

There is safety in numbers.

Any post of honour is a post of great danger.

Custom makes all things easy.

So many people, so many opinions.

Two wrongs do not make one right.

Two is company, three is a crowd.

Cognitive dissonance inhibits the collective mindmode.

Do not punish the innocent
in order to prevent criminals to escape punishment.

An unceremonious person needs great talent to succeed.

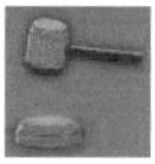

Every person for themselves.

If there were no receivers, there would be no thieves.

Lie down with dogs, wake up with fleas.

People who are their own lawyers have fools for clients.

Protect the chain of command.

Collective thinking fosters morality.

Bad friends prevent you from having good friends.

Human laws should not discriminate.

Give fools enough rope and they will hang themselves.

If people never fear death,
how could the use of executions scare them?
If people always fear death and act abnormal,
how could I dare
to seize, hold, and execute them [1] §74?

A stagnated law is broken by revolution.

Straws tell which way the wind blows.

No one should be judge in his own case.

No person can serve two masters.

Too many cooks spoil the broth.

An oppressive collective weakens,
because it inhibits inventions.

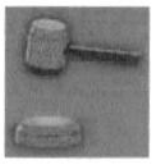

Do not fight with someone who has nothing to lose.

When followers want nothing,
then their leader should fear everything.

Revolutionaries should be very concerned
about what will follow their revolution.

Rules increase the content of the law
and, therefore, there will be more criminals [1] §57.

Never make an empty threat,
because it only warns your opponents.

Revolutions are not made with rosewater.

Human laws deliver order, rather than justice.

Use your collective mindmode
in combination with
your objective, creative, and reactive mindmodes.

It is a sin to steal a pin.

Who pays the piper calls the tune.

The rabble is not influenced by reason, but blind impulse.

The law applies equally to all.

Many hands make light work.

When you buy friends with anything
other than friendship,
they do not stay bought long.

Happy is the country without history.

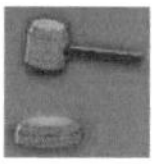

Human law should be blind.

The more prohibitions there are in the world,
the poorer the people will be.
The more sharp weapons people have,
the more the State's household
will be confused [1] §57.

Live and let live.

We must convince by reason, not enforce with dogmas.

Delegate until you have enough spare time to manage.

No greater cruelty
than administered under the collective banner of justice.

A person who cannot obey cannot command.

Blood is thicker than water.

Do not take their dwellings by force.
Do not reject them a place to live.
Only, if they are not rejected,
they will not reject you [1] §72.

It takes two to make a quarrel.

One law for the rich and one for the poor.

Allowing small offences will foster large offences.

Do not do to others
what you do not want them to do to you.

Power corrupts and absolute power corrupts absolutely.

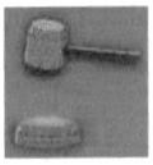

Two heads are better than one.

Collective thinking fosters law and order.

If the world possesses the Way,
then racehorses will be kept for their manure.
If the world is without the Way,
then warhorses will be bred in the suburbs [1] §46.

One beats the bush, while another catches the birds.

Every law has a loophole.

In ruling, the goodness is order [1] §8.

If you want to live and thrive, let the spider run alive.

No one is guilty before the verdict.

Nothing is more noble than politeness,
and nothing more ridiculous than ceremony.

Politics makes strange bedfellows.

Pursue justice, rather than justifications.

People are known by the company they keep.

Misfortune is easier to bear, if shared with many.

A friend to all is a friend to none.

Not enforcing human law is punishing law-abiding people.

If no agreement is reached, then separate.

The highest branch is not the safest roost.

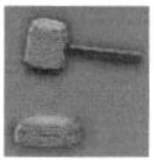

Other times, other manners.

Use the Way to assist the leaders of people.
Do not use soldiers to force the world.
Such actions are likely to rebound [1] §30.

Misfortune reveals those
who only pretend to be your friends.

Human's temporary rules
are subject to nature's eternal laws.

Do not perish to save someone else.

Those who act
on behalf of the one that is in charge of the executions,
execute as if they act on behalf of the Master Carpenter.
From those who act on behalf of the Master Carpenter
only a few will not cut their hands [1] §74.

An eye for an eye and a tooth for a tooth.

Meddle in affairs of others
and to the end of life there will be no safety [1] §52.

Practice Non-action
and the people will transform themselves [1] §57.

What people will do with you, they will do against you.

The insight of a friend is better than good wishes.

Like father like son.

One person may steal a horse,
while another may not look over the hedge.

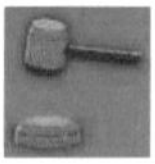

Respect others,
because they are descendants of survivors.

Divide and rule.

Treat your friends with care,
because they might become your enemies.

Armies are the tools of misfortune.
Therefore, armies are not
the tools of great people [1] §31.

Those complying against their will
are of their own opinion still.

Punishment should balance the crime.

Those who wear embroidered coloured silk,
carry sharp swords, gorge on food,
and have a surplus of goods and resources,
are called 'boasting thieves' [1] §53.

Wrong things remain wrong,
even if done for the right reason.

If the great Way is rejected,
then there will be benevolence and justice.
Knowledge and cleverness will appear
and then there is great hypocrisy [1] §18.

The quality of a leader is determined
by the quality of his advisers.

Make the weak strong
so that they can carry their own weight.

An enemy will agree, but a friend may argue.

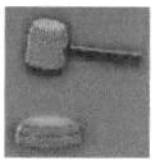

Those who travel alone travel fast.

A friend in need is a friend indeed.

Those who have propriety
possess only a thin layer of loyalty and sincerity,
which is the beginning of disorder [1] §38.

Who cannot be ruled by the rudder
will be ruled by the rock.

Leaders who run out of bribes, are forced to use force.

Those who desire to lead people
must place themselves behind them.
Therefore, they stay above
and the people will not weight them down.
They stay in front
and the people will not harm them [1] §66.
Who lives with the sword will die by the sword.

Do as you would be done by.

Act with Non-action,
then there will be no anarchy [1] §3.

One may steal a horse,
while another may not look over a hedge.

Use no effort
and the people will become
wealthy by themselves [1] §57.

Good fences make good neighbours.

If you cannot beat them, then join them.

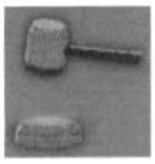

Failing laws will catch the small and free the large.

A bad compromise is better than a good lawsuit.

Sages adhere to orthodox agreements
and do not obligate other people by purpose.
Therefore, those with virtue will uphold the agreement.
Those without virtue will uphold the details [1] §79.

Great leaders are those known by their subjects to exist.
Next are those who are loved and praised.
Next are those who are feared.
Next are those low ones who are insulting [1] §17.

People are hungry,
because their food taxes are high.
Therefore, they are hungry.
Common people cannot be governed,
because their leaders act for their own purposes. Therefore,
the people cannot be governed [1] §75.

Apply your collective mindmode to the laws of people.

Competent warriors do not like war.
Competent chiefs will not get angry.
Competent conquerors will not engage.
Competent leaders will take a low position.
That is called the virtue of not striving [1] §68.

Asking friends to give more
than what they would give voluntarily
is an abuse of friendship.

To know all is to forgive all.

Where ignorance is bliss, it is folly to be wise.

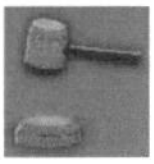

With a king it is the same as with fire;
stay neither too close nor too far away.

A permissive collective weakens,
because it loses direction.

Superior benevolence acts
and yet there is no use in those actions.
Superior justice acts
and there is purpose in those actions.
Superior propriety acts
and if there is no agreement,
then the arms are bared [1] §38.

Favour and disgrace are just like distress [1] §13.

If one wants to take the world,
then one should always use no effort.
When effort is needed,
then there is never enough to take the world [1] §48.

Attack with sharp weapons to become victorious,
but use them without satisfaction.
Those who are satisfied by them,
like to kill people.
Those who like to kill people
cannot achieve the goals of the State [1] §31.

If one sheep leaps over the ditch, then the rest will follow.

Ignorance of the law is no legal defence.

The King is a peasant in the eyes of the law.

Like breeds like.

Focus on behaviour, rather than rhetoric.

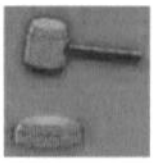

A person who has two enemies must agree with one.

Sages do not strive.
Therefore, no one can strive with them [1] §22.

That someone else is hated
does not mean that you are loved.

No reward should be satisfying,
because that removes the dependency on further rewards.

Those in a large country
only desire to merge and raise people.
Those in a small country
only desire to join other business people.
They all obtain what they desire.
Therefore, the larger one better acts
as the lowest one [1] §61.

Exception proves the rule.

The weakness of democracy
is an incompetent population.
The weakness of dictatorship
is an incompetent leader.

Birds of a feather flock together.

Honey catches more flies than vinegar.

A chain is as strong as its weakest link.

Be just, before you are generous.

Human laws should not be retrospective.

Let him stay at the oar who has learnt to row.

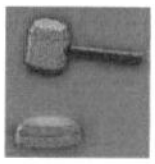

You scratch my back and I will scratch yours.

In an established organisation,
titles will appear.
If titles appear,
then know that it is time to stop.
Know when to stop
and there will be no danger [1] §32.

There is no little enemy.

Armies are the tools of misfortune.
They are disgusting.
Therefore, those who possess the Way
will not claim them [1] §30.

Sages keep their friends close and their enemies closer.

One hand for yourself and one for the ship.

Punishment backfires always.

There is no normal.
Normal turns around and becomes abnormal.
Good turns around and becomes evil [1] §58.

Culture changes the beast into a human.

Do not be pathetic by demanding ceremony at all cost.

Take beggars to court and you will catch only fleas.

One volunteer is worth two pressed men.

Return property to its owner,
and your sleep will be peaceful.

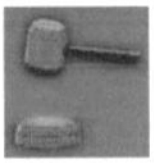

Fish always stinks from the head downwards.

Leaders have to use either manipulation or force.

Do not value knowledge
and the people will not strive.
Do not admire goods
that are difficult to obtain
and the people will not steal.
Do not display
what is desirable
and the people will not revolt [1] §3.

Never ever reward disrespect.

If the laws are very lax,
then the people will have extreme surpluses.
If the laws are very strict,
then the people will have
extreme shortages and misfortune [1] §58.

Left wing or right wing, it is the same bird.

Meddling in the business of others
allows them to meddle in yours.

Judge not, so that you not be judged.

No person is above or below the law.

There is an exception to every law.

Sages will rule for the stomach and not for the eyes.
Therefore, reject that and accept this [1] §12.

The law governs people,
while reason should govern the law.

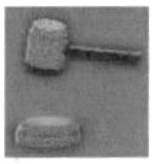

A person who touches pitch shall be defiled.

Fish always stinks from the head downwards.

Leaders have to use either manipulation or force.Discard
adoration and reject knowledge
and the people will benefit a hundred times.
Discard benevolence and reject righteousness
and the people will return to filial piety and compassion.
Discard cleverness and reject profit
and there will be no burglars and thieves [1] §19.

Lend your money to a friend and you will lose a friend.

Uneasy lies the head that wears a crown.

The Way of Nature is not to strive,
but to overcome through competence [1] §73.

Councils of war never fight.

Collective thinking should foster justice.

**A collective without wisdom
is counterproductive.**

Creative

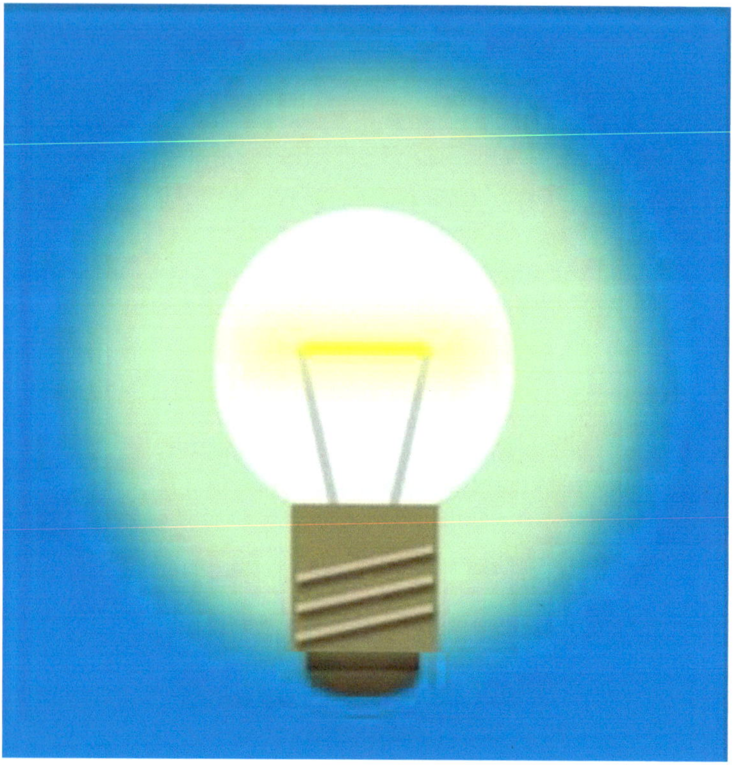

Mantra: I search for ideas.

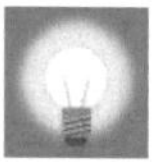

Description Creative

Creative is the nemonik that prompts your mind to generate creative affecters such as innovations and ideas.

The more people know, the stranger the things they begin to develop [1] §57. Creative refers to unreal descriptions of reality. The creative mindmode uses subconscious affectorial thinking in order to deal with the future and the unknown aspects of reality. However, creative affecters could be too unrealistic, illogical, and unreasonable to be applied.

Strength—creative thinking fosters ideas and inventions that deal with the future, the unique, and the unknown.

Weakness—creative thinking is part of affectorial thinking, rather than rational thinking. Therefore, many ideas and inventions are unrealistic, illogical, and unreasonable.

Opportunity—creative thinking could foster progress and deal with nonfactual problems.

Threat—creative thinking could foster the destruction of the planet and humanity. Many ideas and inventions have created manmade extinction problems and are used to kill people. It is a thin line between creativity and insanity.

Wisdom relevant to Creative

An idea is not right just because it is yours.
An idea is not wrong just because it is not yours.

Ideas arrive with early daylight.

Creativity comes in leaps and bounces.

Static opinions inhibit dynamic creativity.

Creativity is the most valuable asset of any organisation.

Innovation is fuel for technology.

A good idea remains a good idea; even if it is not yours.

You can only be exceptional if you deviate from normal.

Use your creative mindmode to cope with the unknown.

It is only creative if it is different.
If it is different it will be criticised.

Do not repeat things that fail.

Dynamic thinkers search for patterns.

Tradition and creativity
are as far apart as solid ice and liquid water.

External and internal brainstorms foster creativity.

Create ideas by synthesizing ideas.

Do not inhibit your creative mindmode with criticism.

Thirty spokes merge into one hub,
but its Nonexistence is useful for a carriage.
Moulded clay makes a cup,
but the Nonexistence of clay is useful for a cup.
Chiselled doors and windows make a room,
but their Nonexistence is useful for a room.
Therefore, using Existence is beneficial,
while using Nonexistence is useful [1] §11.

Generate ideas by applying
collective thinking to the artificial problems.

The more people know,
the stranger the things they begin to develop [1] §57.

Evaluate your ideas afterwards with common sense.

A silent mind fosters creativity.

Create ideas by synthesizing components.

Groupthink inhibits the creative mindmode.

Be patient, because creativity takes time.

Conscious effort kills creativity.

Creativity needs mental freedom.

Dynamic thinkers challenge dogmas.

Generate ideas by considering
focus, balance, efficiency, and proactivity.

Create ideas by dividing entireties.

Write unused ideas down for later.

Dynamic thinkers
believe that they can change anything they want.

You have to break the mould in order to create a new one.

Creativity is the father of science.

Dynamic thinkers evaluate
both differences and similarities.

Sleep fosters creativity.

Create ideas by connecting the dots.

Use your creative mindmode
in combination with your
objective, collective, and reactive mindmodes.

Do not keep repeating things that fail.

Dynamic thinkers turn things upside down.

If your ideas are not different,
then they are not important.

Dynamic thinkers challenge groupthink.

Generate them and raise them.
Generate, but do not possess [1] §10.

Rational thinking makes incremental steps,
while creativity makes quantum leaps.

Dynamic thinkers oppose
their own cognitive dissonance.

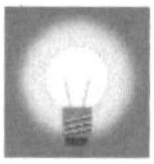

An idle mind fosters creativity.

Relying too much on old ideas inhibits new ones.

You might have lost your creativity,
but you were born with it.

Many great ideas appear to be irrational at the beginning.

The immutable rules of logic inhibit creativity.

Only new ideas can solve old problems.

If mud is settled, stir it
and then it will slowly come alive [1] §15.

If your ideas stop flowing, then take a break.

Show internal gratitude
when your creative subconscious
presents ideas to your conscious.

The creative mindmode
is subconscious and affectorial.

Dynamic thinkers
dream about the impossible.

Think outside the box.

Generate ideas by applying
reactive thinking to repetitive problems.

Generate ideas by considering
to advance, stay, and retreat.

Activate your creative mindmode by asking questions.

One good idea might pay for the rest of your life.

Generate ideas by applying
objective thinking to the natural problems.

Creativity sets people apart from computers.

Create ideas by questioning beliefs.

If everyone in the world recognises
beauty as beautiful,
then there is already ugliness [1] §2.

Trusting your inner genius will foster your creativity.

Generate ideas by considering
to act, wait, and prepare.

Generate ideas by applying
creative thinking to unique problems.

Do not wait for inspiration, just start creating.

Good ideas are accepted willingly,
while bad ideas have to be forced upon people.

Cognitive dissonance inhibits the creative mindmode.

Creativity is a precious jewel that cost you nothing.

Fight a writer's block by writing.

The devil's advocate is a creative devil.

Leave criticizing your ideas to other people.

Punishing mistakes will inhibit creativity.

Each idea has an incubation period.

Nemonik thinking is systematic creativity.

Generate ideas by considering
to accumulate, preserve, and dispose resources.

Start with the solution
and work backwards to the problem.

Laziness is the creative attitude.

Necessity is the mother of invention.

Recalling the twenty-one nemoniks one-by-one
will activate your creative mindmode.

Tune into the creativity of your inner child.

A mindless task fosters creativity.

Ideas are affecters
produced by your subconscious creative mindmode.

Criticism inhibits creativity

Generate ideas by considering
to reveal and conceal things.

Dynamic thinkers
swap causes with symptoms and vice versa.

Generate ideas by considering
to accept and reject things.

The Way is empty,
but use it and it has not to be refilled [1] §4.

Dynamic thinkers challenge the status quo.

The creative mindmode is active during twilight.

Creativity is the hallmark of a genius.

The Way generated the One.
The One generated the Two.
The Two generated the Three.
The Three generated All-things [1] §42.

Nurture creativity with positivism.

Ninety per cent of inspiration is perspiration.

Control inhibits creativity.

The world's things originate from Existence.
Existence originates from Nonexistence [1] §40.

Relaxation fosters creativity.

Word association fosters creativity.

Do not inhibit your creative mindmode with logic.

The Way generates All-things and raises them [1] §51.

Dynamic thinkers evaluate
both what is available and what is lacking.

**Creativity without wisdom
is counterproductive.**

Reactive

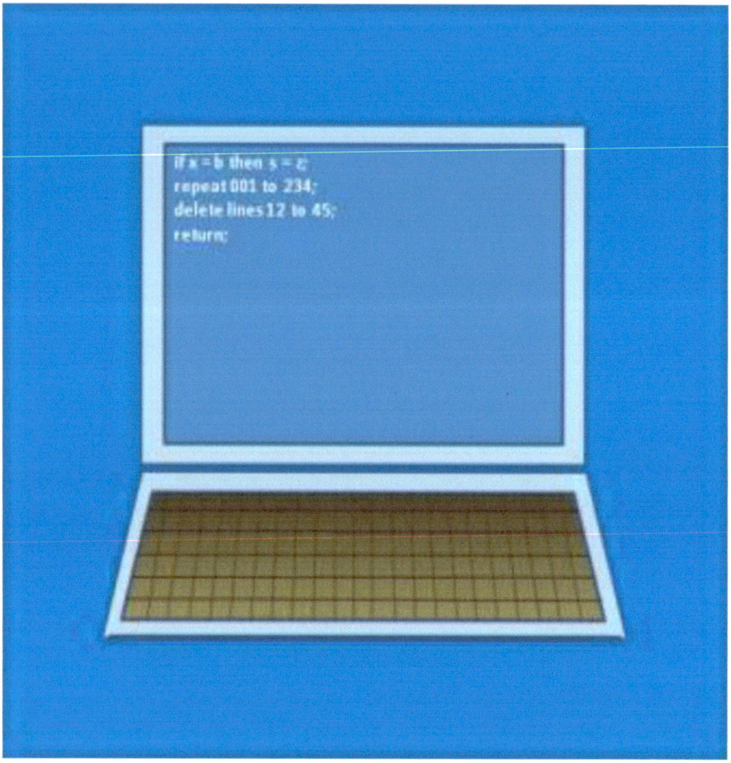

Mantra: I trust my genius.

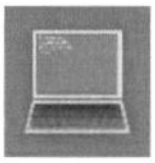

Description Reactive

Reactive is the nemonik that prompts your mind to generate reactive affecters such as emotions, feelings, and skills.

Listening to many details is exhausting and not as good as following your heart [1] §79. Using the subconscious reactive mindmode involves affectorial thinking, the silent mind, and the hidden genius. Your reactive mindmode takes full advantage of your talents, experience, and skills.

Strength—reactive thinking fosters your fastest and most accurate response possible at any given time. All repeated tasks are turned into mindsets that produce reactive affecters.

Weakness—reactive thinking evokes counterproductive reactions (e.g. anger and violence). Therefore, one has to improve the reactive mindmode with Mind Management.

Opportunity—reactive thinking could foster productive habits and perfection.

Threat—reactive thinking could foster counterproductive habits and failure.

Wisdom relevant to Reactive

The conscious might consider,
but the subconscious decides.

Manage your subconscious
otherwise you subconscious will manage you.

Worrying is not thinking.

Foster serenity to accept
the things you cannot change.

Foster the courage to change
the things you should change.

Those who use compassion
to attack will triumph [1] §67.

Hate is a bad adviser.

Foster the wisdom to know
the difference between the possible and impossible.

Our subconscious determines the quality of our lives.
It sends our conscious either good or bad affecters.

Mental firewalls prevent you
to change the beliefs of others.

One dies
the way one lives.

All mental suffering is created by the sufferer.

Use your reactive mindmode
in combination with
the objective, collective, and creative mindmodes.

Let the dead take care of the dead.

No conflict is more counterproductive
than between the conscious and subconscious.

Fear is the killer of the little mind.

Only those who have internal balance
can inhibit external conflicts.

Intuition might be wrong but it never lies.

When the going gets tough, the tough get going.

The heart has reasons that reason does not understand.

Hate is a fire that will consume you.

If you suffer look inside.

Love is a game that two play and both can win.

Anxiety that has no root in reality
is counterproductive.

Our subconscious creates and rules our reality.

Inhibiting the reactive mindmode
demotes the master to a novice.

The subconscious makes the conscious suffer.

If there is conflict then look inside for the solution.

Our conscious has no choice,
but to live in harmony with our subconscious.

Those who remember the past
will be always at war.

Do not try to put new wine into old bottles.

All suffering is self-inflicted.

If you miss love, then you miss life.

Better to have loved and lost,
than never to have loved at all.

Our subconscious can create
a multitude of illusionary demons
that ruin our lives for no reason.

Those who are compassionate
can be courageous.
Those who are frugal
can be generous.
Those who are humble
can be successful leaders of affairs [1] §67.

Sages are not weak.
They consider their weakness as a weakness.
Hence, it is not a weakness [1] §71.

Those who see anxiety as an outside problem
will never get rid of it.

Envy will suffocate your soul.

Pride goes before the fall.

Suffering is an imbalance
between our conscious and subconscious.

Acts of kindness may soon be forgotten,
but the memory of an offense remains.

If passion drives, let reason hold the reins.

Forgive and forget; or hate will ruin your life.

Improve your subconscious with mantras
and you will improve your life.

Trust your subconscious,
because it is much larger than your conscious.

Wilful people will have their way.

Reason is absent when impulse rules.

Never send a novice to do a master's job.

One who always jokes is a joker.

Arrogance causes misfortune [1] §16.

Let not the sun go down on your anger.

Sages have always three treasures
that they keep and protect.
The first one is called compassion.
The second one is called frugality.
The third one is called humbleness [1] §67.

The noblest vengeance is to forgive.

Those who stand on tiptoe do not stand firm [1] §24.

Who gets angry without reason,
makes peace without satisfaction.

A snake can lose its skin,
but it still remains a snake.

In ruling people and working with nature
there is nothing like frugality.
Only those who are frugal
are called to early service [1] §59.

Envy remembers the faults of others,
rather than their greatness.

A savage temper makes all things a crime.

Practice makes perfect.

Those who keep the Way do not desire fullness.
Only those who desire no fullness
are therefore able to exhaust themselves
without renewal [1] §15.

Never underestimate your opponents,
because they descent from survivors.

You cannot teach an old dog new tricks.

Young people think that old people are fools,
but old people know that young people are fools.

Once bitten, twice shy.

Your mental firewall protects your correct beliefs,
but also your incorrect ones.

Punctuality is the politeness of kings.

A person who cannot tolerate small misfortunes
can never accomplish great things.

Do not cry about spilt milk.

Sages do not boast about themselves.
Therefore, they have merit [1] §22.

The novice repeats again and again
in order to become a master.

Know your own faults before blaming others for theirs.

Do not blame bullies,
because if you reward a child for winning inside the class,
then that child will also try to win outside the class.

Follow your heart, but check where you go with your head.

Greater qualities are needed
to bear good fortune than bad.

Fools try to change the concrete outer reality,
while sages change the plastic inner reality.

If you believe in God
then you have to become the best you can be
to please the highest power.
If you do not believe in God
then you have to become the best you can be,
because you are the highest power.

A burnt child dreads the fire.

Reactivity is the best available response at any moment.

Night brings counsel.

What is past cannot be prevented
and should not be grieved for.

It is not work that kills, but stress.

Hope springs eternal.

Cleanse your heart from greed,
and your feet remain free from shackles.

Plant positive seeds in your mind.

Love will find a way.

Reactivity fosters survival in emergencies.

A person who slowly gets angry
will stay angry for a long time.

Despite all conscious reasoning,
the subconscious reactive mindmode decides.

A stout heart overcomes ill fortune.

Admiring wealth and arrogance
brings personal loss and misfortune [1] §9.

Experience is the father of wisdom.

Do not look for logic in intuition.

No matter how thoroughly a crow may wash,
it remains forever black.

Arrows pierce the body, while words pierce the heart.

The novice acts, while the master reacts.

Subconscious reaction is superior to conscious action.

Those who are arrogant are without development.
Their Way is callcd:
Leftover food and unnecessary action [1] §24.

We soon believe what we desire to believe.

A belief is an accepted,
but untested description of reality.

Expertise is stored in the reactive mindmode.

The reactive mindmode creates your inner reality.

A drowning person will soon learn to swim.

Making a choice between hope and fear
is emotional, rather than rational.

The head works hard, while the heart works smart.

The teachers of humanity
discuss and teach people
that violent people
will achieve nothing but death [1] §42.

Mindsets are subconscious sets of rules or algorithms
that generate affecters.

Who goes to Rome a beast returns a beast.

The leopard cannot change his spots.

Logic only proves what intuition already knows.

What cannot be cured must be endured.

People learn little from success, but much from failure.

All things are difficult before they become easy.

A fool at forty is a fool indeed.

Love is blind.

Those who overcome other people have power.
Those who overcome themselves are strong [1] §33.

You cannot be in love and be wise at the same time.

Civility cost nothing.

Using the mind's vital energy
is called powerful [1] §55.

In an emergency, rely on your reactive mindmode.

Patience is a flower that grows not in everyone's garden.

The eyes are the windows to the soul.

Where passion reigns there is no room for reason.

Cognitive dissonance inhibits the reactive mindmode.

People who live in hope dance to a bad tune.

Belief begins where reason stops.

The heart determines whether the head is believed.

Old habits die hard.

Repay hatred with kindness [1] §63.

If you cannot be good, be careful.

Discard adoration and reject knowledge
and the people will benefit a hundred times.
Discard benevolence and reject righteousness
and the people will return to filial piety and compassion.
Discard cleverness and reject profit
and there will be no burglars and thieves [1] §19.

Zeal without knowledge is a runaway horse.

It is easier to prevent ill habits than to break them.

Those who are courageous in daring
will be killed.
Those who are courageous in not daring
will live [1] §73.

Sages are not arrogant.
Therefore, they will develop [1] §22.

Genius is an infinite capacity for taking pains.

Logic inhibits intuition.

Apply your reactive mindmode to repetitive problems.

Pain is an affecter that warns you about damage.

Intuition provides no explanations, but only directions.

A fruit bearing tree is known by its flowers.

The reactive mindmode is subconscious and affectorial.

A mental firewall protects
the subconscious information against change.

Act with a silent mind. Act without thinking.

Learn to think on your feet.

Intuition knows before the head computes.

If it were not for hope, the heart would break.

An empty mind is a silent mind.

Personal growth is based on repetition.

Trust the genius that lives in your reactive mindmode.

Self-confidence is two-thirds of success.

Fear is the antidote for pride.

Little things please little minds.

Intuition is seeing without thinking.

Your beliefs are frozen by your mental firewall
whether they are correct or incorrect.

Each belief is perceived by the owner
as an immutable fact.

Cowards die many times before their deaths.

Reject your subconscious genius often
and it will stop trying to get your conscious attention.

There is no fool like an old fool.

Only those who do not act for the purpose of living
are knowledgeable at valuing life [1] §75.

You are always right;
whether you tell yourself that you can
or that you cannot.

Let the dead bury the dead.

Things that should be forgotten
are most easily remembered.

Learn how to swim before you go near the water.

It is harder to conquer yourself than the world.

Acting from stubbornness is inviting disaster.

You learn from what does not kill you.

Strive for inner perfection,
then the outer perfection takes care of itself.

Habituation is the tool
to improve your reactive mindmode.

Past behaviour predicts future behaviour.

Lack selfishness and restrain desires [1] §19.

Wash a dog, comb a dog, and still a dog remains a dog.

If you fill your head with pride
you will lack space for wisdom.

Fear is a double-edged sword
that protects with warnings and kills with panic.

The hand that rocks the cradle rules the world.

You are the only one who can improve your belief-system.

Experience is the best teacher.

No greater suffering
than having extreme desires.
No greater misfortune
than not knowing what is enough.
No misfortune is more disastrous
than the desire to accumulate.
Therefore, know that enough is enough
and there will be always enough [1] §46.

You cannot put an old head on young shoulders.

There is no greater misfortune,
than being unable to endure misfortune.

If you are not a flower, then do not be a thorn.

One hour sleep before midnight is worth two hours after.

Passion is an energy to be used carefully.

Know yourself.

If you do what you always did,
you will always remain what you always were.

You never know what you can do until you try.

Focus on either happiness or sadness; the choice is yours.

If words change your emotions,
then someone is pushing your buttons.

An ounce of practice is worth a pound of instructions.

Increase your mindpower by repeating your mantras.

Those who are arrogant
are without development [1] §22.

In thinking, the goodness is depth [1] §8.

The reactive mind
is like a garden that needs constant weeding.

You are only young once,
but you can stay immature indefinitely.

Sages desire not to desire and do not admire goods
that are difficult to obtain [1] §64.

Some fail because they feel everything,
others fail because they feel nothing.

Where there is a will there is a way.

Mantras are signals from the conscious
aiming to improve the subconscious.

Extreme mental firewalls make people
either gullible or stubborn.

To err is human and to forgive is divine.

Do not pride over your wealth or beauty,
one will be gone in a night and the other with a fever.

Your mind controls your reality.

Think as the best thinker you could be.

Kindness is free.

Pride and grace dwell never in the same mind.

Affecters are signals from the subconscious
aiming to manage the conscious.

There is no better company in a scrap than a brave heart.

Bewitch others with courtesy.

Those who have desires will not succeed [1] §24.

Listening to many details is exhausting
and not as good as following your heart [1] §5.

Stay always calm, cool, and collected.

The reactive mindmode is the storehouse of your skills.

A guilty conscious does not need an accuser.

None so blind as those who do not want to see.

Politeness and honour are free for you to give
and priceless for others to receive.

Groupthink inhibits the reactive mindmode.

Those who abandon compassion
and are yet courageous;
abandon their frugality
and are yet generous;
abandon their humbleness
and are yet leading;
they will certainly die [1] §67.

All common people focus their ears and eyes.
Instead, all sages are like children [1] §49.

Sudden passions throw prudence of balance.

The reactive mindmode is the superior mindmode.

Succeed without boasting.
Succeed without attacking.
Succeed without arrogance.
Succeed without excess [1] §30.

It is never too late to learn.

Those who know other people are wise.
Those who know themselves are brilliant [1] §33.

Reactivity without wisdom
is counterproductive.

Advance

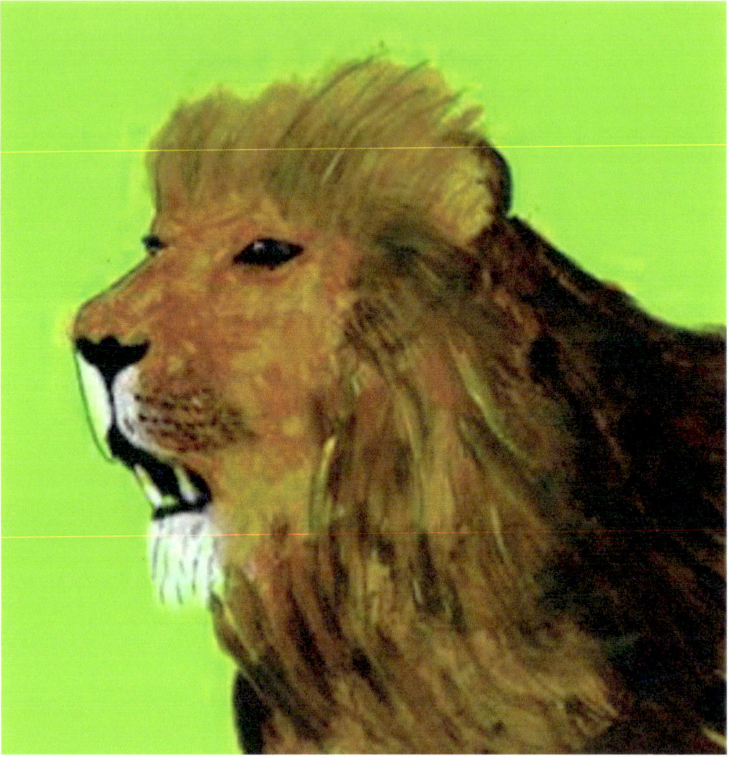

Mantra: I advance to where I can stay.

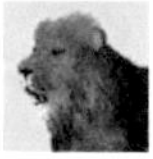

Description Advance

Advance is the nemonik that prompts your mind to decrease the distance to your goal.

I do not dare to advance an inch, but retreat a foot [1] §69. Advance only to positions where you can stay. Otherwise, you will lose time and resources in the futile advance and the subsequent forced retreat. Examples of ignoring this rule are the failed campaigns in Russia of Napoleon (1812) and Hitler (1941). Neither of them could stay in Moscow.

Strength—advancing moves you closer to the realization of your goal.

Weakness—advancing increases the length of your supply lines.

Opportunity—advancing could create a fast momentum that creates chaos and unbalances your opponents. An advance could surprise your opponents, give you the initiative, and provide new resources.

Threat—advancing could lead you into unknown territory and traps. Therefore, scouting the unknown territory is crucial.

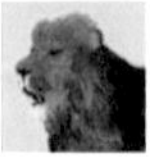

Wisdom relevant to Advance

An overextended advance is a weak advance.

Those who use compassion
to attack will triumph [1] §67.

Don't advance too far
if you have to return the same distance.

Keep up with the times, do not stay in the dark.

When your enemies retreat, make them a golden bridge.

Surprise, concentration, and speed
will strengthen your advance.

Prepare your advance thoroughly.

The aim of advance is to move closer to your goal.

Create a vacuum to advance into.

Attack is the best defence.

Make sure that you neutralize enemy strongholds
that you leave behind.

If you take big paces then you leave big spaces.

Use all available natural and artificial forces
in your advance.

It is easier to advance with a sail than a paddle.

A journey of a thousand miles begins with a single step.

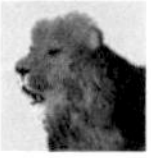

Maintain the speed of your advance
by bypassing obstacles.

A person who does not advance recedes.

No progress without struggle.

Advancing gives you the initiative.

He who doesn't look ahead stays behind.

Make sure that your advance does not run out of steam.

There is no advance without a goal.

Extend your territory through an advance.

Whether you advance quickly or slowly,
the distance remains the same.

Sages maintain the momentum of their advance.

There is always room at the top.

Advancing will cost you resources.

Not every movement is an advance.

Advance without disturbing the balance.

There is no advance without change.

A superior advance is unpredictable.

Advancing downhill adds gravity to your momentum.

Slow but sure wins the race.

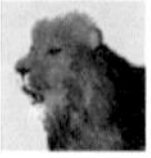

Sages do not stretch their resources
too thin during their advance.

Those who advance have to leave where they are.

Sages never start a fight that they cannot win.

Be wary to advance when your opponent retreats.

Preserve your supply lines when you advance.

If you have a thesis, then advance to the antithesis.

When you advance, focus on your advance.

The Way forward seems to be backwards [1] §41.

You may advance when your opponent retreats.

One step at the time.

Sages give their opponents an easy way to retreat.

Focus your greatest strength on the greatest weakness.

Align your advance with forces that restore the balance.

If you advance,
then consolidate first what you have achieved already.

Advance holds the threat of entering unknown territory.

Use your opponent's retreat to advance without effort.

Sages never spur a willing horse.

An advance may accumulate resources.

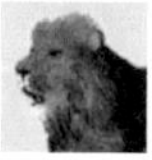

The success of an advance depends on its focus.

Not all advance is progress.

If you have an antithesis, then advance to the synthesis.

Do not advance if you cannot complete it.

Stay a while, and lose a mile.

Surprise is at the core of a strong advance.

When water stays for long it stinks.

If you advance, then be aware of ambushes.

Advance only to places where you can stay.

Use a vacuum to advance,
because nature abhors a vacuum.

Consider the reactions before you advance.

Create a deviation to cover your advance.

Use the spoils of your advance,
to support your advance.

A person who stays in the valley,
shall never get over the hill.

There is no advance without risk.

One gets lice by staying in the same place.

Be wary if you advance in response to a challenge.

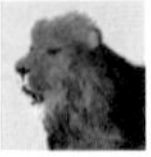

Be cautious for traps
if your advance meets no resistance.

Progress is to escape what you suffer.

Incompetent people
advance to their level of incompetence.

Confuse your opponent before you advance.

Flowing water never gets dirty.

Advancing is moving towards your goal.

Progress is to obtain what you seek.

Progress without a goal is madness.

During your advance,
do not give your opponent time to regroup.

Maintain your formation during your advance.

Attack with sharp weapons to become victorious,
but use them without satisfaction.
Those who are satisfied by them,
like to kill people.
Those who like to kill people
cannot achieve the goals of the State [1] §31.

An apparently easy advance may lead you into a trap.

Sages do not advance straight into a stonewall.

Advancing is moving away from your suffering.

Progress requires a dynamic mind.

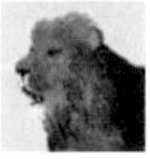

Those who stay where no profit is found,
remain fools the whole year round.

Sages advance only after they have considered
to stay and retreat.

Advance focussed and efficiently.

The secret to success is to walk forwards.

**Advancing without wisdom
is counterproductive.**

Stay

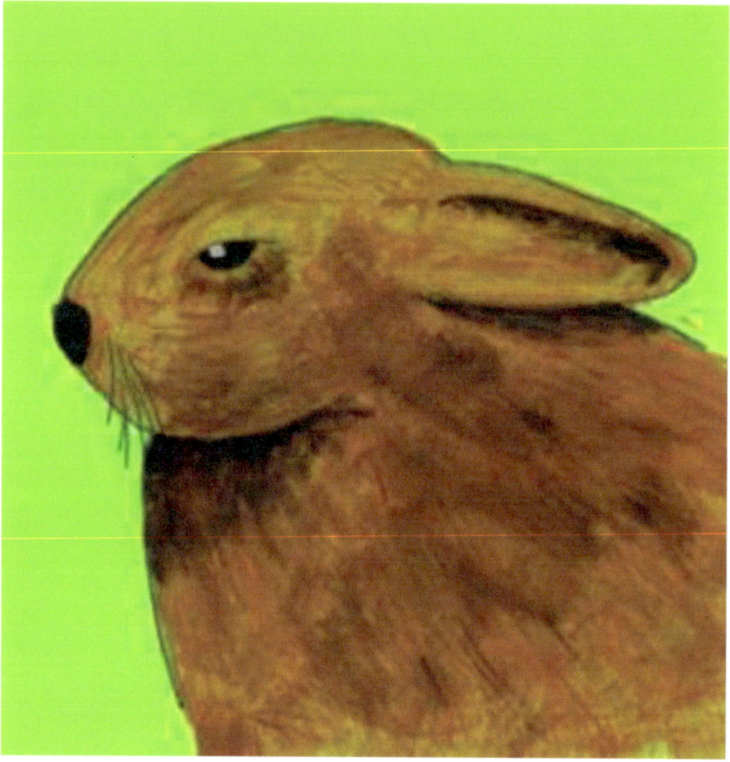

Mantra: I stay where I can leave.

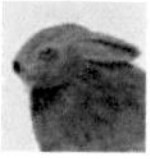

Description Stay

Stay is the nemonik that prompts your mind to maintain the same distance to your goal.

Those who use the Way of Nature (Physics) to defend will stand firm [1] §67. Stay only in positions from where you can retreat. Examples of ignoring this rule are the sieges of the Jewish fortress Masada by the Romans (73) and the Alamo during the war between the Texan revolutionaries and Mexico (1836). Lacking the possibility to retreat, all defenders perished.

Strength—staying protects previous advances.

Weakness—staying losing the initiative, momentum, and surprise.

Opportunity—staying could foster recuperation and regrouping.

Threat—staying could foster the predictability of your future actions. It could also foster isolation, immobility, and depleted supplies. Your opponents might bypass, besiege, break through, and surround your position.

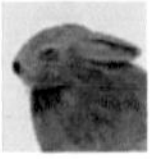

Wisdom relevant to Stay

If you stay at home you won't wear out your shoes.

To lose your ability to move
is a threat of staying in one place.

Stay, because out of sight out of mind.

Stay where there are songs.

When a bull refuses to move,
you cannot make it go ahead
by pulling it by the reins and using your whip.

Who has moved for three times has lived through fire.

To be surrounded is a threat of staying in one place.

If you leave your place, then you lose it.

Waves come and go,
but the ocean stays.

A tree does not move unless there is wind.

An often-moving person
never thrives as well as one that settles down.

The chicken that stays in the farmyard,
will peck the crumbs.

Those who can stay will obtain.

Stay, because the absent person is always in the wrong.

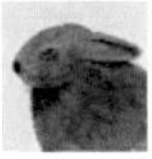

Often moved stones gather no moss.

The stone will not move from its place
unless head is put to head.

There is no winter for who stays in his mother's womb.

One who is not moved by words
is not moved by the stick either.

When staying in someone's home,
leave your defects at the door.

If the wind does not blow, the leaves do not move.

Stay continuously in the vegetable and flower garden.

Life is so short we must move very slowly.

The boat sails by, but the shore stays.

Though the wind blows, the mountain stays.

There is no stay without risk.

Choose your lodging before dark
and leave before the morning dew.

You cannot hold another fellow down in a ditch
unless you stay down there with him.

Do not leave the high road for a short cut.

War does not determine who is right, but who stays.

If your part of the battlefield is covered with thorns,
do not leave your position.

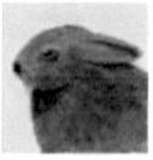

Water that has reached its level does not flow.

There is courage in opposing suggestions

for a too rash advance.

Stones will stay forever, while water passes.

It is better to be sorry and stay,
than to be sorry and go away.

If a frog leaves the swamp for the mountains,
it means it is in danger.

When you leave home,
you do not know who will feed you.

A rolling stone gathers no moss.

Speak highly of the lake, but stay on the bank.

Succeed without attacking [1] §30.

If you sit on a comfortable seat, do not leave that seat.

A person who moves fast through life
has no place to call home.

Losing the initiative
is a weakness of staying in one place.

Three kinds of people die poor:
those who divorce,
those who incur debts,
and those who move around too much.

Water flows, but rocks stay.

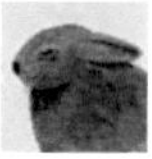

Those who are discontent
to remain in one place
will not earn much.

Stay only after you have considered
to advance and retreat.

Sages stay only at places from where they can leave.

People are divided into three classes:
those that are immovable,
those that are moveable,
and those that move.

Quiet rivers have flowery banks.

Let him who is well off stay where he is.

Stay a little and the job will finish quicker.

A sandstorm passes; the stars remain.

Yielding prolongs war.

When you stay, focus on your staying.

Although shrimps dance around,
they do not leave the river.

That what comes to stay cannot return.

A person who makes the first bad move,
always loses the game.

Stay,
because when the cat is away
the mice will play.

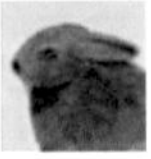

Plants often moved never thrive.

Business goes where it is invited
and stays where it is well treated.

To be happy, stay at home.

If you stay long enough in one place
the whole world passes by.

Destroy a country,
but still its mountains and rivers stay.

Prudent stays make speedy journeys.

Consolidating your position is a strength of staying.

Better not to move at all than do so and regret it.

Do not leave the betrodden way for the untrodden one.

A wind can move the branches of trees,
but it will never move the head of a wise person.

When people move away from nature,
their hearts become hard.

Stay a little and news will find you.

The wise traveller leaves his heart at home.

Go further and fare worse.

When all the water has gone,
only the largest stones will stay on the riverbed.

Technological advance fosters humanity's extinction.

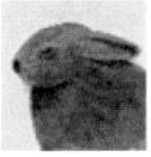

To leave a place is to die a little.

A person who can sit upon a stone
and feed himself should not move.

The cat has nine lives:
three for playing,
three for straying,
three for staying.

Those who are competent
succeed and stop in time [1] §30.

A prospering person remains at home.

When the earth is hot, the worm stays in the ground.

Do not stay in a place
from where you cannot move away.

If the wolf had stayed in the woods
then there would have been no hue and cry after him.

A person who travels a lot becomes wise.
A person who stays home is wise.

A chameleon does not leave one tree
until he is sure of another one.

The sage and the tortoise may travel,
but they never leave their homes.

Staying without wisdom
is counterproductive.

Retreat

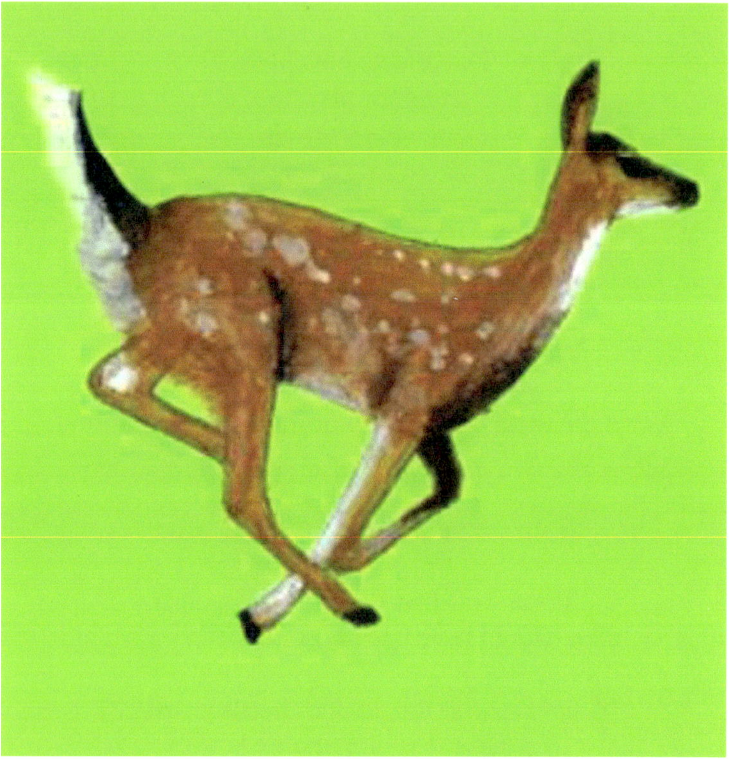

Mantra: I retreat to where I can stay.

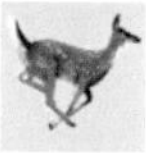

Description Retreat

Retreat is the nemonik that prompts your mind to increase the distance to your goal.

I do not dare to advance an inch, but retreat a foot [1] §69. A retreat is not a defeat. Examples are Mikhail Kutuzov (1812) and Joseph Stalin (1941) who retreated from respectively Napoleon and Hitler. By retreating, they used the harsh climate, scorched earth, and an overextension of the enemy supply lines to their advantage.

Strength—retreat fosters the preservation of your life and resources.

Weakness—retreat moves you away from your goal.

Opportunity—retreat could return you to known territory comprising safety, and resources. It could be a strategy of scorched earth, that reduces your supply lines, extend the supply lines of opponents, and lure your opponents into unknown territory. You could regroup, resupply, and set traps. Retreat is no defeat.

Threat—retreat could create a chaotic rout leading to defeat.

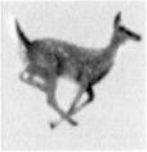

Wisdom relevant to Retreat

Better to flee and stay alive than to die a hero.

Do not let your retreat turn into a chaotic rout.

Retreat in glory,
because applause at your entrance
is not based on your performance.

Defuse your opponent's advance with retreat.

Retreat is just another strategy to maximize your success.

When merit is achieved,
withdrawing yourself is the Way of Nature [1] §9.

It is no disgrace
to move out of the way of a charging elephant.
Returning to the roots is called tranquillity.
Tranquillity is called returning to order.
Returning to order is a constant.
Knowing this constant is brilliant.
Ignoring this constant is arrogant [1] §16.

Retreat to a place from where you can leave.

When you retreat, focus on your retreat.

Returning is the movement of the Way [1] §40.

Absence makes the heart grow fonder.

A cat in a corner will fight.

Retreating is not the same as fleeing.

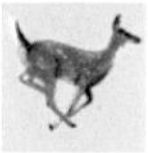

Every time the Way returns to Nothingness [1] §14.

Youth may stray afar yet they return at last.

A person who rides a tiger is afraid to dismount.

Rats leave a sinking ship.

Be wary when things have reached their top.

A good retreat is better than a poor advance.

A person who leaves and then returns, had a good trip.

Retreat only after you have considered
to advance and stay.

Better to be a living dog than a dead lion.

All-things around us rise,
and I watch them return.
Those things are numerous
and each one returns to its roots [1] §16.

Where you have left without a quarrel
is where you are about to return.

Sages withdraw themselves. Yet they are first [1] §7.

A superior retreat may overcome the opponent's advance.

Many cowards would retreat if they had courage enough.

Even far away things return to the Way [1] §65.

It is easier to hide from danger than to face it.

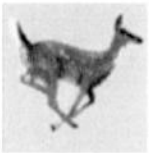

The bird flies high, but always returns to earth.

Advancing or staying does not exclude a future retreat.

Let a rear-guard protect your retreat.

Great means continuous.
Continuous means forever.
Forever means returning [1] §25.

I do not dare to act as a host,
but act as a guest.
I do not dare to advance an inch,
but retreat a foot.
That is called:
moving without moving.
Rolling up the sleeves
without showing an arm [1] §69.

Sages retreat to a place where they can stay.

Retreat faster than your opponent can advance.

It is better to flee than to remain in disgrace.

There is no retreat without risk.

Bend then be preserved.
Twist then be straightened [1] §22.

A failed advance may force a catastrophic retreat.

All-things return to the Way [1] §34.

A constant guest is never welcome.

Quit while you are ahead.

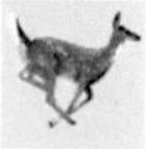

On the way out, the road is rough;
on returning, the road is smooth.

Fleeing is shameful, but it preserves your life.

Fish and guests stink after three days.

Better bend than break.

The threat of any retreat is a chaotic rout.

When two people quarrel;
the one who yields first,
displays the nobler character.

Fight only when you can win; retreat when you cannot.

Fallen leaves return to the root.

Run away to fight another day.

If the eternal virtue never leaves,
then you will return to infancy.
If the eternal virtue never errs,
then it returns to moderation.
If the eternal virtue is always enough,
then you will return to simplicity [1] §28.

Returning to known territory is a strength of retreat.

Those who fight and run away, live to fight another day.

No matter how much you feed a wolf,
he will always return to the forest.

One must draw back in order to leap.

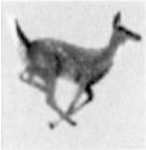

Retreat in order to advance.

Retreat is no defeat.

Better return half way than lose everything.

If you cannot stand the heat, then get out of the kitchen.

Keep your formation intact during a retreat.

Those who bend will be preserved [1] §22.

Better to return halfway
than to continue on the wrong road.

Let the people return
to knotted cords and use them [1] §80.

Mice always return to their own little holes.

Any port in a storm.

Better retreat in honour than advance in disgrace.

Set ambushes to protect your retreat.

Only the dead never return.

It is better to return from the centre of the ford
than to drown in the flood.

**Retreating without wisdom
is counterproductive.**

Accumulate

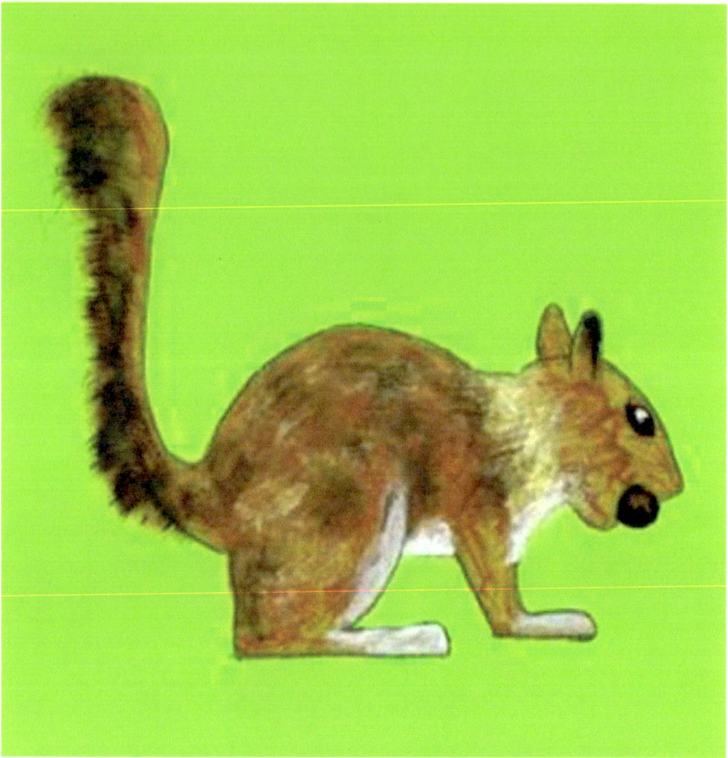

Mantra: I accumulate productive resources.

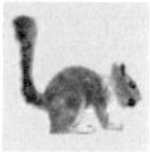

Description Accumulate

Accumulate is the nemonik that prompts your mind to increase the amount of matter that is under your control.

No misfortune is more disastrous than the desire to accumulate. Know that enough is enough and there will be always enough [1] §46. Accumulation for the sake of accumulation is counterproductive. Instead, maintain your focus and accumulate only those resources that are needed to maximize your success.

Strength—accumulating increases your safety buffer.

Weakness—accumulating increases the preservation cost.

Opportunity—accumulating could foster strategic options, comfort, and freedom.

Threat—accumulating could foster accumulation for the sake of accumulation. The tool could become the goal fostering greed and hoarding. That could foster the possibility to become a public target. *A room filled with gold and jade cannot be defended competently* [1] §9.

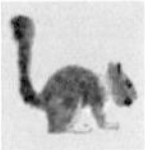

Wisdom relevant to Accumulate

One person's trash is another person's treasure.

Accumulate a thing of beauty
and you accumulate a joy forever.

Where a river flows there is abundance.

Acquired knowledge inhibits acquiring knowledge.

Keep company with people who make you look good.

The reason that some people are stingy
is also the reason that they are rich.

You might as well be hanged for a sheep as for a lamb.

Acknowledging ignorance
starts the accumulation of knowledge.

Those who go borrowing go sorrowing.

An empty purse frightens away friends.

The vultures are where the carcass is.

Money has no smell.

Don't mistake your wants for your needs.

The worth of a thing is best known by the want of it.

Catch as catch can.

No money—no life.

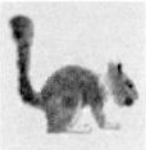

Whether it is drugs, money, or fame; people have lost themselves if their desires have become needs.

A heavy purse makes a light heart.

The sea refuses no river.

What's yours is mine and what's mine is my own.

Do not accumulate only a single resource;
no matter how precious.

Nobody has ever bet enough on a winning horse.

Money is power.

Never buy a pig in a bag.

Those who do not learn from the past
will have to learn from war.

All is fish that comes to the net.

I use no effort
and the people will become wealthy
by themselves [1] §57.

Walnuts and pears you plant for your heirs.

Accumulate goodwill by providing goodwill.

Fools build houses and sages live in them.

You can't buy happiness.

People who watch their fortune grow
find their houses too small.

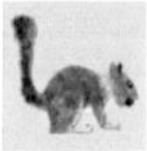

Accumulate resources only after you have considered
to preserve and dispose them.

Misfortune is fortune's place to hide [1] §58.

You cannot make an omelette without breaking eggs.

Something is better than nothing.

The wise learn from the past.
The ignorant just repeat it.

It is good fishing in troubled waters.

Fair exchange is no robbery.

Little by little and bit by bit makes a mountain.

A little rain each day will fill the rivers to overflowing.

Beggars cannot be choosers.

A golden key opens every door.

Money talks.

Speculate to accumulate.

An early person never borrows from a late one.

A successful person accumulates the right supporters.

Fair flowers do not remain long by the wayside.

Accumulate beneficial things,
rather than pleasurable ones.

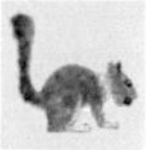

Beauty is in the eye of the beholder.

To get what you want,
you must accept some things you do not want.

Do not accept payment in politeness.

Don't pay for something you want
with something you need.

There is no accumulation without risk.

What is between the Sky and the Earth
is like a pair of bellows.
It is empty, but not exhausted.
Use it and more will be produced [1] §5.

Know the successful in order to join them
and know the unsuccessful in order to avoid them.

Listening provides what you do not know.

When the Emperor is crowned
and the three ministers are installed,
a millstone of jade preceded by four horses,
is not as good as sitting down
and presenting this [1] §62.

Fortune is always on the side of large battalions.

Associate with the successful.

Fortune gives many too much, but no one enough.

When you accumulate, focus on your accumulation.

Poverty is no disgrace, but it is a great inconvenience.

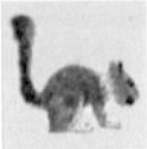

Half a loaf is better than no bread.

Fortune knocks at least once at each person's gate.

Where there is muck there is gold.

Accumulate without effort.

One's loss is another's gain.

Money begets money.

Fine feathers make fine birds.

Quick returns make rich merchants.

The best fish swim near the bottom.

Industry is the parent of fortune.

Where bees are, there is honey.

Every little bit helps.

Small winnings make a heavy purse.

Every person has a price.

Comfort is better than pride.

Don't swap something you need
for something you want.

Better be envied than pitied.

Much wants always more.

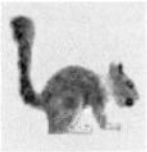

Buy in the cheapest market
and sell in the dearest.

What is disposed by others
can be accumulated without cost.

From the same flower
the bee extracts honey and the wasp gall.

The remaining fish in the sea
are as good as ever came out of it.

Little and often fills the purse.

Finders keepers and losers weepers.

The buyer needs a hundred eyes, the seller only one.

Big fish eat little fish.

Out of debt, out of danger.

Accumulating without wisdom
is counterproductive.

Preserve

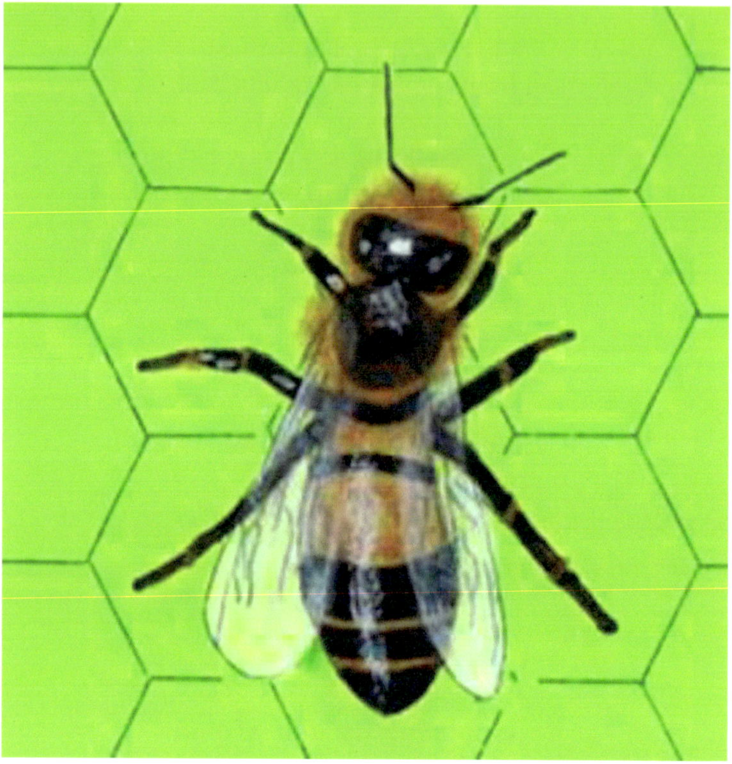

Mantra: I preserve accumulated resources.

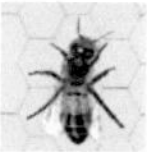

Description Preserve

Preserve is the nemonik that prompts your mind to maintain the same amount of matter that is under your control.

A room filled with gold and jade cannot be defended competently [1] §9. It is counterproductive to accumulate resources without preserving them. However, preservation demands effort and resources, because everything is subject to a gradual decline or entropy. Hence, the preservation of many resources will cost many resources.

Strength—preservation protects your previous efforts and investments in the accumulation of your resources.

Weakness—preservation increases the cost of preservation and reduces the amount of accumulated resources. It is counterproductive to preserve what should be disposed.

Opportunity—preservation could maintain your strategic options.

Threat—preservation could destroy your resources through decay or entropy.

Wisdom relevant to Preserve

Pleasing words might be exchanged.
Respectful conduct might honour people.
Incompetent people
forsake their Existence unnecessarily [1] §62.

Whether the jug strikes the stone, or the stone the jug,
it is bad for the jug.

Preserve your support network by honouring
your father and mother.

Remember past success in order to create future success.

Destroy the gunners, but preserve the guns.

Do not pour out the dirty water before you have clean.

Even as the archer loves the arrow that flies,
so too he loves the bow that remains in his hands.

The eye is bigger than the belly.

Preserve resources only after you have considered
to accumulate and dispose them.

Keep a thing seven years and you will find a use for it.

Any port in a storm.

Do not desire the great splendour of jade,
but the grace of natural rock [1] §39.

Greed creates counterproductive imbalances.

It is never too late to mend.

Never look a gift horse in the mouth.

Better safe than sorry,

What you have, hold.

A rich person has not a lot, but instead needs little.

Those who are competent have not much.
Those who have much are not competent [1] §81.

Willful waste makes sorrowful wants.

A penny saved is a penny earned.

Those who live in glass houses should not throw stones.

Dirty water will still quench fire.

Those who are frugal can be generous [1] §67.

Save well and you will have resources to spend.

Those who know what is enough are rich [1] §33.

It is much easier to fall in love than to stay in love.

Half a loaf is better than no bread.

Fools never notice the water until the well is dry.

An old poacher makes the best gamekeeper.

Do not cast pearls before swine.

Something is better than nothing.

Best to be on the safe side.

While there is life there is hope.

Waste not, want not.

You have to lie in the bed you make.

Some day you might value
what seems to be worthless right now.

The more things change,
the more they remain the same.

Kill not the goose that lays golden eggs.

An army marches on its stomach.

Little leaks sink big ships.

Bend then be preserved [1] §22.

Know that enough is enough
and there will be always enough [1] §46.

Burn not your house to fright the mouse away.

Keep something for a rainy day.

Prices are soon forgotten, quality remains.

Incompetent people
know only the value of the things they lost.

Gluttony kills more than the sword.

You cannot preserve your cake and eat it.

So long as the green mountains are preserved,
there will be no shortage of firewood.

Preserve not what should be disposed.

Accumulating and filling up
are not as good as stopping in time [1] §9.

You cannot dispose the cow and still drink the milk.

There's many a good tune played on an old fiddle.

Incompetent people know always the cost of things,
but never their value.

One courts misfortune by flaunting wealth.

Those who bend will be preserved [1] §22.

Gold may be bought too costly.

Do not accumulate what cannot be preserved.

Know what is enough
and there will be no disgrace.
Know when to stop
and there will be no danger.
Accordingly, one will endure long [1] §44.

If people give to you, they expect more in return.

Money is like the water of a river flowing away.

It is a foolish bird that soils its own nest.

Call in great favours only for great occasions.

One's name remains above the grave.

Do not risk your reputation on one roll of the dice.

Rhinoceroses have no place to ram their horns.
Tigers have no place to strike their claws.
Soldiers have no place to thrust their swords.
What is the reason?
Because sages avoid the realm of death [1] §50.

What is loaned goes away smiling but returns weeping.

A room filled with gold and jade
cannot be defended competently [1] §9.

A bird in the hand is better than ten in the air.

Keeping is harder than winning.

When you preserve, focus on your preservation.

Thrift is a great revenue.

No greater misfortune
than not knowing what is enough [1] §46.

Aphorisms are preserved wisdom.

Spread your eggs over many baskets.

Enough is as good as a feast.

Beauty passes; wisdom remains.

Do not throw out the baby with the bathwater.

Do not change horses midstream.

A creaking door hangs longest.

Emerging into life is entering into death.
Three in ten are companions of life.
Three in ten are companions of death.
Three in ten people live extremely
and move into the realm of death [1] §50.

What is worth accumulating is worth preserving.

Opportunity makes a thief.

Hold on to what you have.

Health is more valuable than wealth.

Do not walk through the hills
in order to meet rhinoceroses and tigers.
Do not join the army
in order to carry weapons [1] §50.

A good name is sooner lost than won.

Some people live extremely.
They are incompetent
in hiding, listening, and conserving their lives [1] §50.

Fixing the known is better than waiting for the unknown.

Let the people be serious about death
and not move far away [1] §80.

It is easier to destroy than to build.

Do not dispose what you might need tomorrow.

He is rich who has few wants.

Give too much too soon,
and people fall in love with your hand,
rather than your heart.

To have two eyes is cause for pride;
but to have one eye is better than to have none.

A person in debt becomes a slave.

Have surplus then be confused [1] §22.

If people always fear death and act abnormal,
how could I dare
to seize, hold, and execute them [1] §74)?

Keep something in reserve for setbacks.

Life or wealth?
What is worth more?
Gain or loss?
What hurts more?
Most people love to spend a lot.
The larger their hoard
the more they have to lose [1] §44.

Do not cut off your nose to spite your face.

Sages save people always competently
by not rejecting them.
Not rejected things are resources [1] §27.

What is fated to be yours will always return to you.

An old tree will die if shifted.

Money is like air, you do not notice it unless it is gone.

Fortune has a fickle heart
and soon asks back what it has given.

Grasp all, lose all.

People who repair not their gutters
have to repair their whole house.

Proverbs are preserved parts of minds.

Preservation without wisdom
is counterproductive.

Dispose

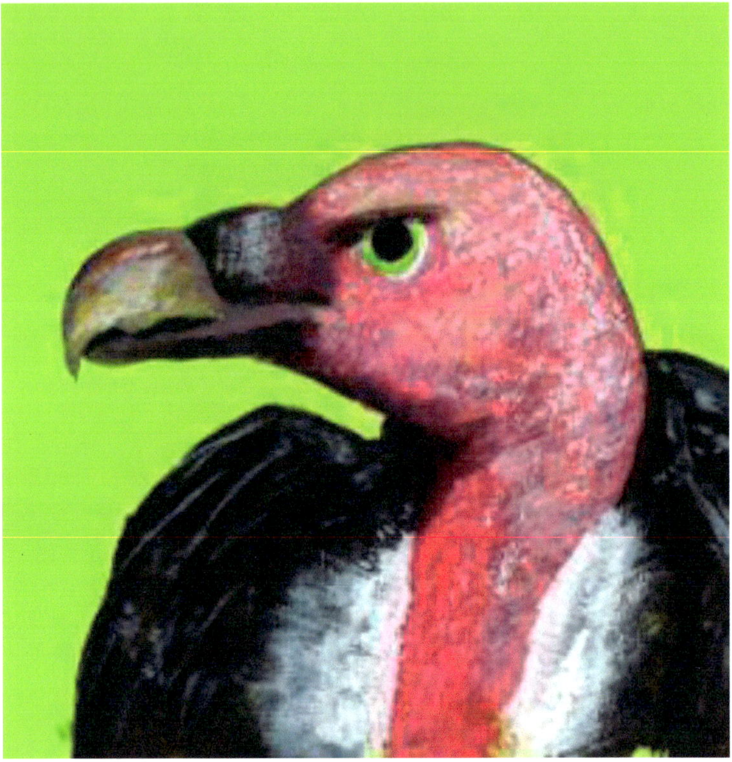

Mantra: I dispose unproductive resources.

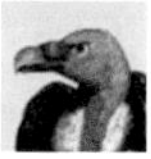

Description Dispose

Dispose is the nemonik that prompts your mind to decrease the amount of matter that is under your control.

Those who hold will lose [1] §29. The larger their hoard the more they have to lose [1] §44. Sometimes a person has to dispose resources in order to maximize his or her success. For example, if lost in the Kalahari Desert it is counterproductive to carry fifty kilos of gold. Maximize your success by disposing the extra weight.

Strength—disposal decreases the preservation costs of your resources.

Weakness—disposal causes the loss of investments and costs associated with the earlier accumulation and the preservation of those resources.

Opportunity—disposal could increase your mobility and decrease the mobility of your opponents. You might dispose resources in order to set a trap (Trojan Horse). As they say: *Beware of Greeks bearing gifts.*

Threat—disposal could cause shortages in the future.

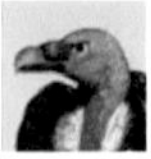

Wisdom relevant to Dispose

It is useless to flog a dead horse.

The rotten apple injures its neighbours.

A light purse makes a heavy heart.

What a neighbour gets is not lost.

Give quickly and you give twice.

Knowledge decays.

Discard knowledge
and there are no worries [1] §19.

Too many cooks spoil the broth.

Friends suffer so that their friends
maximize their success.

Clipped porcelain never breaks.

Sages reject extremes,
reject grandeur,
and reject extravagance [1] §29.

Hang on tightly and let go lightly.

Throw out a sprat to catch a mackerel.

That which leaks cannot stay full.

What costs nothing is worth nothing.

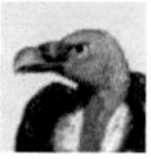

A person with a full purse has many friends.

Let bygones be bygones.

A bit of fragrance clings to the hand that gives flowers.

Who owns too much, remains unhappy.

Not all the flowers of a tree produce fruit.

Fallen blossoms do not return to branches.

Those who always preserve their reputations,
can never effect a reform.

Those who put business before friends
have no real friends.

Payback is a bitch.

The sun loses nothing by shining into a puddle.

The need to dispose of a friend
is the result of accumulating that friend.

Do not dispose too easy of friends.

Sages do not hoard.
Since they are used to act for other people,
they receive more possessions for themselves.
Since they are used to give to other people,
they have much more themselves [1] §81.

Soon ripe, soon rotten.

Do not dispose your soul.
You will have to live with it.

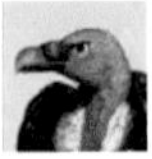

A promise made is a debt unpaid.

Do not defend your ideas like they are your babies,
but advance and find the next one.

Many things are more pleasurable
when they belong to others.

Generate, but do not possess [1] §10.

If friends have no wings, then they are imperfect.

You cannot lose what you never had.

You must lose a fly to catch a trout.

Wilful waste makes woeful want.

Once you have made a fortune, know how to spend it.

You can have too much of a good thing.

A person who waits to be asked, gives too late.

You cannot make an omelette without breaking eggs.

You cannot dispose what you never had.

Let the water you cannot drink flow by.

It is an ill bird that fouls its own nest.

Consider the shortcomings of your friends as ugly faces.
Just look deeper.

A superior gift
requires deep knowledge of the receiver's needs.

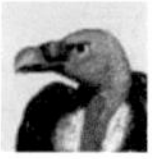

Like flowers, gifts please most when they are fresh.

Give fools enough rope and they will hang himself.

Give and take is fair play.

Ill weeds grow fast.

Give a dog a bad name and hang him.

Those who have plenty
and give to those in the world who have not enough
are the only ones who possess the Way [1] §77.

More than enough is too much.

If a stone is thrown at you,
throw back some bread in return.

Bees touch no fading flowers.

If people always fear certain death,
then there is always someone in charge
of executing them.
Those who act on behalf
of the one that is in charge of the executions,
execute as if they act on behalf
of the Master Carpenter.
From those who act
on behalf of the Master Carpenter
only a few will not cut their hands [1] §74.

You cannot get blood from a stone.

The bigger they are, the harder they fall.

The past is water under the bridge.

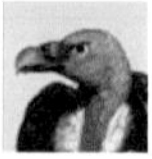

There's a black sheep in every flock.

Ill-gotten goods never thrive.

A bad penny always comes back.

Easy come easy go.

Charity begins at home.

Those who are not part of the solution
are part of the problem.

Only a fool will not dispose a fool.

Bad money drives out good money.

The love of money is the root of all evil.

Those who draw their sword against the prince
throw their scabbard away.

Let beauty scatter the mirror in time.

The best of friends must part.

Even the fairest rose will wither.

When in doubt leave it out.

All good things come to an end.

No imbalance can be maintained forever.

Dispose resources only after you have considered
to accumulate and preserve them.

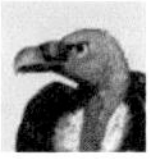

Lightly come, lightly go.

Everything has its time.

Put a beggar on horseback, and he will ride to the devil.

A tree that doesn't flower in April, won't flower at all.

Let the left hand not know what the right hand is doing.

A useless watch dog barks, but stays far away.

Treachery returns.

A broken mirror will not reflect again.

A fool and his money are soon separated.

A few things gained by fraud,
destroy a fortune otherwise honestly won.

Whet their appetites with gifts, but do not overfill them.

Discard adoration and reject knowledge
and the people will benefit a hundred times.
Discard benevolence and reject righteousness
and the people will return to filial piety and compassion.
Discard cleverness and reject profit
and there will be no burglars and thieves [1] §19.

Cut your losses, before your losses cut you.

Do not keep what inhibits your success.

The worth of a thing is what it will fetch on the market.

When you dispose, focus on your disposal.

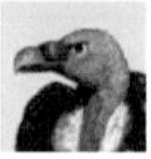

A gift long waited for is sold, not given.

Who gives, teaches a return.

Do not throw away your old shoes
before you have new ones.

Goods given, make quicker return than goods held.

An unwanted thing is expensive at any price.

It is no good to die with redundant resources.

Stolen things bring misfortune.

Shrouds have no pockets.

Even the highest tree has an axe waiting at its foot.

A tiger never returns to his unfinished prey.

**Dispoasal without wisdom
is counterproductive.**

Act

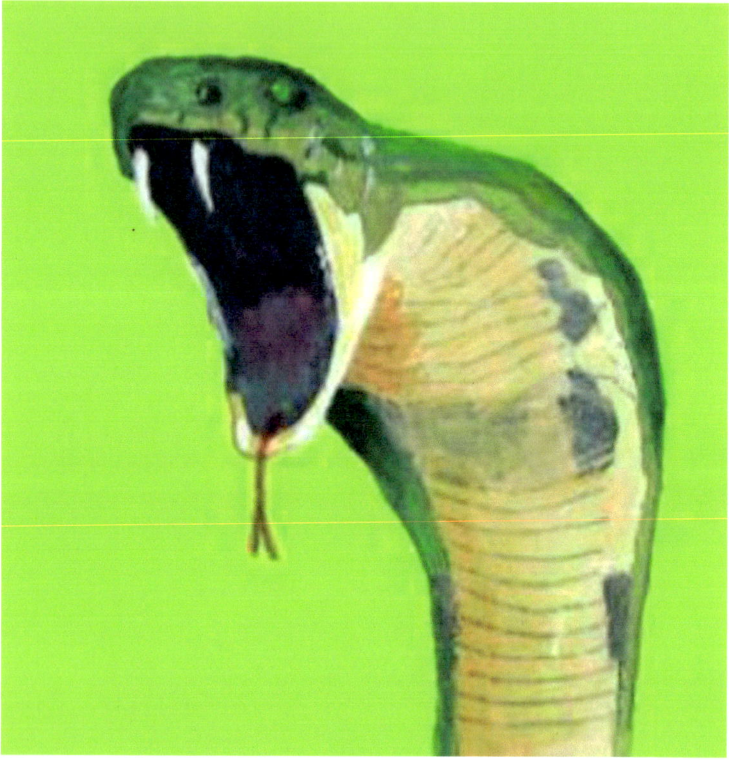

Mantra: I act with determination.

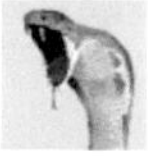

Description Act

Act is the nemonik that prompts your mind to change or move matter in space and time.

When merit is achieved, withdrawing yourself is the Way of Nature (Physics) [1] §9. If you decide to act then decide also when to stop. For example, the US ignored this rule and is now engaged in several long-term wars. Even winning those wars might not anymore maximize the success of the US. If you act, then act with the snake's determination and a silent mind. Give it your all without doubt.

Strength—action turns your ideas into reality.

Weakness—action evokes reactions, which might be larger than the action [3].

Opportunity—action could be proactive and prevent a problem to grow beyond control.

Threat—action could be proactive or reactive. Proactive action could be unnecessary, because the threat did not materialize. On the other hand, reactive action could be too late. In addition, acting rashly in order to reduce the stress and anxiety of waiting for the right moment of action.

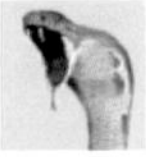

Wisdom relevant to Act

Ensure that your actions
produce productive reactions.

Actions that disturb a balance will be undone.

An action in anger
is an action to regret.

Actions speak
louder than words.

Those who take up the sword
will be destroyed by the sword.

Fortune often knocks at the door,
but fools do not invite her in.

Fools rush in, where angels fear to tread.

Those who act will fail.
Those who hold will lose.
Therefore, sages will use Non-action.
Therefore, they will not fail.
They will not hold.
Therefore, they will not lose [1] §64.

Speedy execution is the mother of good fortune.

Being late is a counterproductive disrespect of others.

Time is money.

Since sages are used to act for other people,
they receive more possessions for themselves [1] §81.

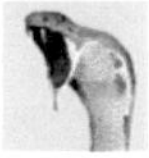

Those who hesitate are lost.

Time does not return.

Unless you act, nothing happens.

Sages do not act and yet they achieve [1] §47.

No time like the present.

It is not how you start.
It is how you finish.

If you wait for an opportunity, then you may wait forever.

You never know what you can do until you try.

Your actions today determine who you will be tomorrow.

Act with Non-action [1] §63.

Who has time and yet waits for time,
comes to a time of regret.

Hoist your sail when the wind is fair.

You could wait till the cows come home.

Time is the most precious commodity.

Only act when the situation will get worse.

Time can be stopped by none.

Wait is a hard word for the hungry.

Politeness is the key to friendship.

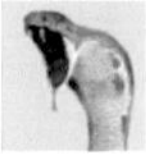

It is the first step that is difficult.

Quickness wins applause.

Foster the courage to change
the things you should change.

People count faults of those who keep them waiting.

Those who are courageous in daring
will be killed.
Those who are courageous in not daring
will live [1] §73.

Preserve the chain of command during action.

If you ever need a helping hand,
you will find one at the end of your arm.

If you snooze you lose.

To maintain your worth,
your words must be backed up by action.

Sages can achieve greatness,
because they do not act great [1] §34.

Time wait for none.

Contract and contract until there is Non-action left.
There is no action and yet there is action [1] §48.

Better to wear out, than to rust out.

Time past never returns.

There is no time like the present.

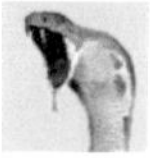

It is childish to remain in a hole
when you can take yourself out.

Opportunity never knocks twice.

People who wait for roast duck
to fly into their mouths must wait forever.

If you think too much about every step,
then you will stand on one leg all your life.

A person who would like to eat the kernel
must crack the nut.

Superior virtue uses Non-action
and there is no action used.
Superior benevolence acts
and yet there is no use in those actions.
Superior justice acts
and there is purpose in those actions.
Superior propriety acts
and if there is no agreement,
then the arms are bared [1] §39.

Fortune favours the brave.

Act with determination.

Make hay when the sun shines.

Each action needs follow-up to the end.

A person who hesitates is lost.

Do not delay until tomorrow what you can do today.

Those who want to eat the fruit must climb the tree.

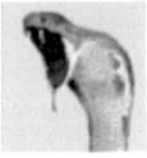

Wait for time and you lose time.

In action, the goodness is timing [1] §8.

Saying is one thing and doing another.

Sages manage their affairs with Non-action [1] §2.

Words might be wise, but actions change the world.

A person of words without deeds
is like a garden full of weeds.

Any dead fish can flow down the river,
but it takes a live one to swim back up stream.

Without action you will never reach your goal.

Take the bull by the horns.

You are what you do, rather than what you say.

A bold attempt is half the success.

Sages act, but do not rely on it [1] §77.

If you wait, you may never start.

Pluck flowers as they bloom;
wait and you'll have only the twigs.

The only thing scary is action [1] §53.

No matter how much snow falls,
it won't remain there all summer.

Deeds count, not words.

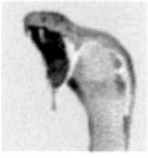

Tide and time wait for no one.

Procrastination kills action.

Never confuse motion with action.

Footprints on the sands of time
are not made by sitting down.

Procrastination is
waiting without a productive reason.

Time is like a river; it flows by and doesn't return.

All waiting is too long.

Act only after you have considered to wait and prepare.

One must fill the jug while the water is flowing.

Procrastination is the thief of time.

Time is money.

In misfortune, people need help, not lamentation.

The world's most difficult things
arise from the easiest.
The world's largest things
arise from the smallest.
Therefore, all sages will avoid great actions [1] §63.

The greatest talkers are the least doers.

Tomorrow never comes.

Waiting harms the stomach.

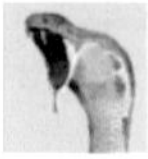

Success is a ladder
which cannot be climbed with hands in your pocket.

If you make the first move
then you have the advantage of being first.

The water of the river flows on
without waiting for the thirsty person.

A wasted day does not return.

Preserve discipline and formation during action.

Fortune does not stand waiting at any one's door.

The dying person cannot wait for the shroud to be woven.

Action without a goal is counterproductive.

When fortune knocks, open the door.

Who can act will act, who cannot act will teach.

First come, first served.

It might be better to ask for forgiveness,
rather than permission.

The first blow is half the battle.

The rambling polecat leaves its house
when there is a banquet.

Life is like a boat:
you move when you paddle and stay if you do not.

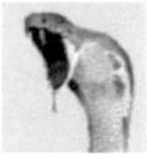

Everything comes to him who does not wait.

Catch the bear before you sell its skin.

I do not dare to act as a host, but act as a guest [1] §69.

One who waits for a chance may wait forever.

Wise people fail through hesitation.

Fortune favours the bold.

The Way of Nature
is beneficial and without harm.
Accordingly, the Way of People
should be action without strive [1] §81.

Nothing ventured, nothing gained.

To him who is determined it remains only to act.

When you act, focus on your action.

In for a penny, in for a pound.

Sages complement the nature of All-things,
but they do not dare to act [1] §64.

If you are lucky then act.

Those who want the fruit must climb the tree.

Those that will not when they may,
when they will shall have nay.

When the food is cooked
there is no need to wait before eating it.

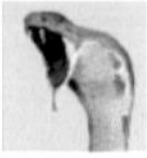

There is no action without risk.

Success and rest do not sleep together.

Only action can turn your dreams into reality.

Sail while the breeze blows,
because wind and tide wait for no one.

No pain, no gain.

Who waits hoping and dreaming,
loses time, and collects flies and troubles.

The softest of the world
will overcome the hardest of the world.
What is without substance
will penetrate what is without gaps.
Therefore, I know that there is benefit in Non-action.
Teaching without speaking and Non-action
will benefit the whole world [1] §43.

Act as the best person you could be.

Feet that are used to move cannot stay.

Though the fool waits, the day does not.

Gather flowers while the morning sun lasts.

Act, but do not rely on it [1] §2, 51.

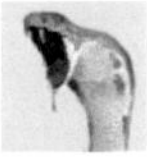

Strike when the iron is hot.

A growing youth has a wolf in his belly.

Action without wisdom
is counterproductive.

Wait

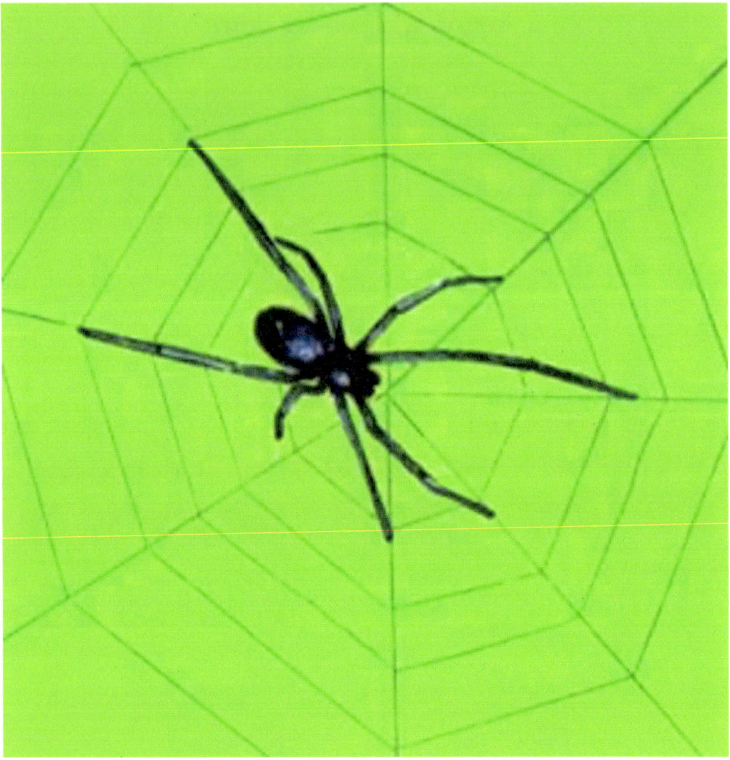

Mantra: I wait for the right time.

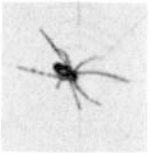

Description Wait

Wait is the nemonik that prompts your mind to delay your action until it is the most productive time for that action.

In action, the goodness is timing [1] §8. Do not act if the situation devclops in your advantage. Go with the flow and let time work for you. However, do not let productive waiting turn into counterproductive procrastination. On the other hand, be proactive if the situation develops in your disadvantage.

Strength—waiting fosters the possibility to act at the most productive time.

Weakness—waiting inhibits your initiative, advance, and momentum.

Opportunity—waiting could work in your advantage if the situation improves. Your opponents might get tense and your waiting might lure them into rash action.

Threat—waiting could work in your disadvantage if the situation deteriorates. Waiting could turn into procrastination.

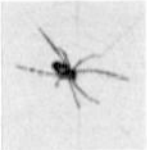

Wisdom relevant to Wait

Wait and let time solve your problem.

Time heals all wounds.

Time is a great problem solver.

Perfection takes time.

Revenge is best served cold.

The praying mantis is never tired waiting all day.

If you wait long enough, it will be good weather.

It is well to stop playing when the game is at its best.

Even the longest day has an end.

Fools fail, because they are always in a hurry.

Wait if time is solving the problem.

Patience soothes many a pang.

Heroes do not die from old age.

Action is silver, waiting is gold.

The spider that knows its gain,
waits patiently in its web.

Each action evokes a reaction
of equal magnitude and opposite direction.

All things come to those who wait.

See what is in the bush
before you throw stones at the noise.

Time works wonders.

Each simple action disturbs a myriad of balances.

One swallow does not make a summer.

Things done cannot be undone.

Hotheadedness
is the shortest way to the executioner's sword.

Hold your horses for the race.

Let him attack who will; the strong wait.

Great oaks grow from a little acorn.

You laugh best when you laugh last.

Rashness is the father of disaster.

You can take a horse to the water,
but you cannot make it drink.

Everything comes to him who waits.

A person who waits shall live to see.

Respond early to every detail
and you will lose momentum.

Procrastination is a thief of time.

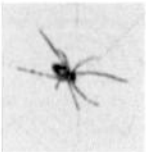

Idle people have the least leisure.

Patience is a virtue.

Those who remove stones rashly
will bruise their fingers.

Wait when the situation gets better

If you find the river flooded, then wait.

Always sleep on it, no matter how urgent.

Haste makes waste.

One flower does not bring spring.

Rashness is the evil twin of proactivity.

Haste is from the Devil.

Better late than never.

Sit on the bank of a river and wait:
Your enemy's corpse will soon float by.

Good things come to those who wait.

Violent rains do not drum all day [1] §23.

Strong things will become weak.
They are not called the Way.
What is not the Way will perish soon [1] §55.

When in doubt—wait.

Sit and wait for the good chestnuts to fall.

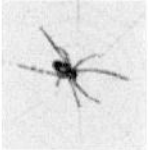

The future is for those who wait.

Waiting lies between wish and reality.

Do not act if you doubt the wisdom of your action.

Make haste slowly.

Do not fill the gap left by a successful person,
because that person cannot make mistakes anymore.

A moment of impatience can ruin your entire life.

Recognize gladly great exploits, but wait a while first.

Many problems are none, if just left alone.

Hold on to the Great Image
and the world will come.
It will come
without harm and with great calm [1] §35.

When you wait, focus on waiting.

Count no person successful until he is dead.

A person who is patient is always successful.

Fortune is like fruit:
if you wait long enough the fruit will fall.

All-things rise, but do not initiate [1] §2.

Wait only after you have considered to act and prepare.

The softest will overcome the hardest.
The weakest will overcome the strongest [1] §78.

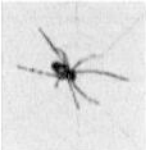

Cast not the first stone.

Haste trips over its own feet.

Given time, a muddy stream will clear.

Avoid rashness, because such action is too early.

Hurry slowly.

Fools do sooner what sages do later.

Those who can wait to prepare
will overcome those who cannot wait to act.

Wait until the tree has fallen, before you jump over it.

More haste is less speed.

The softest of the world
will overcome the hardest of the world.
What is without substance
will penetrate what is without gaps [1] §43.

Fools fail through rashness.

Tomorrow is another day.

Fools rush in where sages fear to tread.

Every action must be executed at the right time.

Those who act will fail.
Those who hold will lose [1] §29.

In action, the goodness is timing [1] §8.

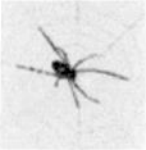

Time is the great healer.

If you wait long enough the world will be your own.

One flower does not make a garland.

Caution helps to achieve success
and console with failure.

What is done immediately will be undone immediately.

Hasty climbers have sudden falls.

Never act, unless it is prudent.

Patient people can have what they will.

Success depends on acting at the right moment.

Sing before breakfast and you will cry before night.

Waiting people get the wind behind them.

Desires are nourished by delays.

Do not count your chickens before they are hatched.

The one who waits for a fine day, will get a fine day.

Do not act just to reduce the tension of waiting.

Patience can conquer destiny.

Hesitation is the child of prudence.

Rashness will lose the sovereign [1] §26.

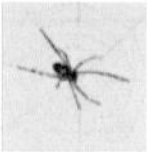

Waiting is delaying action for a productive reason.

Idleness is the root of all evil.

The greatest talent matures late [1] §41.

There is a tide in the affairs of men.

Caution is lacking when it is needed most.

Leave disorder alone and it becomes order.

It is easier to raise the Devil than to lay him down.

You never wait too long
when you wait for something good.

If you would enjoy the fruit, do not pluck the flower.

One who waits patiently will catch a big fish.

A person who can wait obtains what he wishes.

Never show half-finished things to others,
it ruins the surprise.

All fools are bold.

Know when to stop
and there will be no danger [1] §32 & 44.

A little patience can prevent a great disaster.

The musician paid in advance does not play so well.

Without stirring, muddy water will clear.

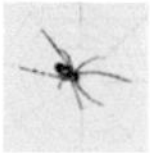

Work paid for in advance has feet of lead.

Rome was not built in a day.

Better safe than sorry.

Time will tell.

Hunger drives the wolf out of the woods.

Early flowers give no seed.

If you are unlucky then wait.

Wait for the night,
before saying that the day has been beautiful.

Wait long, strike fast.

Do not stir mud and it will slowly clear [1] §15.

Do not cross the bridge till you come to it.

Sleep and wait for good luck.

Waiting without wisdom
is counterproductive.

Prepare

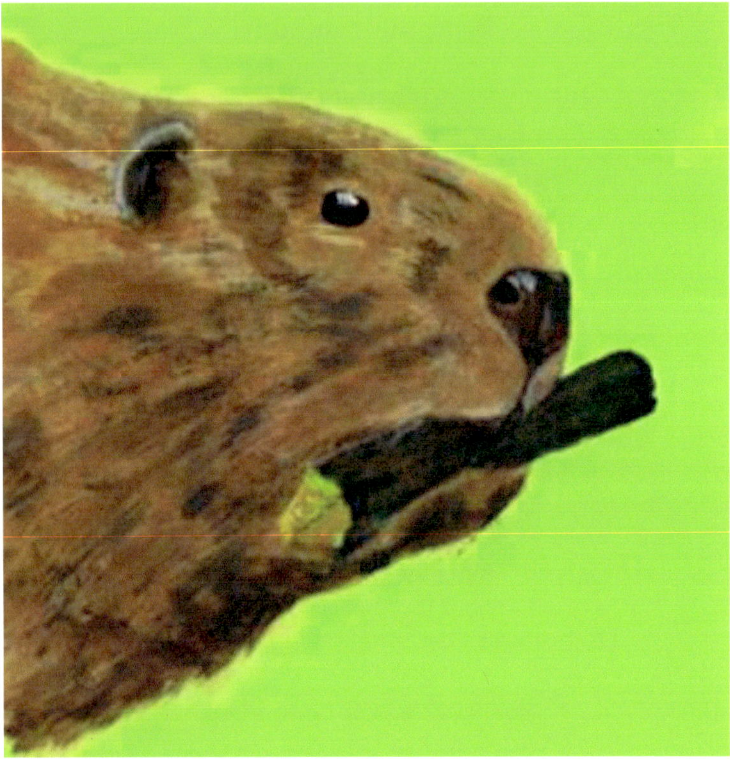

Mantra: I prepare before I wait.

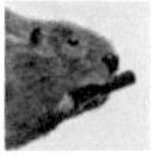

Description Prepare

Prepare is the nemonik that prompts your mind to get ready for your most productive action.

Those who pretend to know the future are the fruitless flowers of the Way of Nature (Physics) and the chiefs of fools [1] §38. Be careful, because you can only prepare for the future if you know that future. Otherwise, preparation might become the counterproductive result of static thinking.

Strength—preparation improves your position.

Weakness—preparation cost resources.

Opportunity—preparation makes the impossible possible.

Threat—preparation could turn into counterproductive procrastination e.g. *paralyses by analyses.* The cost of preparation could be so high that it would cause annihilation (Bankrupt states as result of arms race).

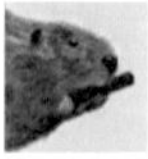

Wisdom relevant to Prepare

Prepare for the next task, rather than the ultimate destiny.

A person who wants to climb the ladder
must begin at the bottom.

No plan is written in stone.

Whatever you sow you will reap.

Preparation is the key to success.

Those who will survive the future,
learn from those who have survived the past.

What could go wrong
will go wrong.

Organise your resources
to be in the right place at the right time.

The road to success is always under construction.

Plan for the future,
because you will spend the rest of your life there.

A diligent person
ever finds that something remains to be done.

Planning reveals pitfalls.

Only if fully prepared,
you can wait for the right time to act.

That what is not manifest is easy to plan [1] §64.

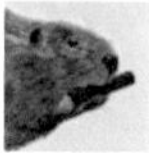

If you are ready,
then you do not have to waste time to get ready.

Well begun is half done.

Plan your life wisely without rushing.

You plant trees for your heirs.

The Way is simple and plans with competence [1] §73.

The unexpected always happens.

Include focus, balance, efficiency, and proactivity
in your plans.

Prepare only after you have considered
to act and wait.

Do not go up a creek without a paddle.

Disorganize your opponent's support network.

Manage the information flow
between your mind and reality.

Planning clears the mind.

Those of value speak about their plans
and succeed in completing their affairs.
Yet, the common people will say;
it happened naturally [1] §17.

Prepare for whatever life could throw at you.

Prepare, rather than waiting unprepared.

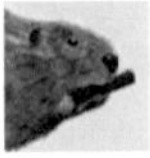

Only the Way
is good at the beginning
and good at the end [1] §41.

Plan diligently,
because you must lie in the bed you make.

Sages win the war before it starts,
because they position themselves in advance.

The best is often the enemy of the good.

All the flowers of tomorrow are in the seeds of today.

It is well to find out from which way the wind blows.

Float a trial balloon and see what happens.

A plan is a dream with a time limit.

History repeats itself.

Cut large tasks into small ones.

The race does not go to the swift,
nor the battle to the strong.

Check all twenty-one nemoniks
for each planned item.

Position yourself before you act.

A good beginning is half the success.

Get your priorities right.

Analyse your situation.

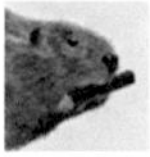

Too early is as bad as too late.

Busy people have ample time.

The pyramids show
that an unmovable mountain can be moved
one rock at the time.

During peace prepare for war.

Focus on one task at the time.

If you want peace; prepare for war.

Plan for failure when successful.

Prepare for the reaction to your action.

Fortune will call at the smiling gate.

Measure twice, but cut once.

If a thing is worth doing it is worth doing well.

Whatever can go wrong will go wrong.

Prepare for the call to serve early
by a significant accumulation of virtue.
If there is a significant accumulation of virtue,
then nothing is impossible [1] §59.

Nothing is so certain as the unexpected.

Analyse the situation of your opponents.

Who stays at the master and does not learn,
is either a fool or pretends to be one.

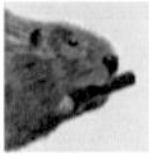

The secret of success is to start from scratch.

Consider the urgency and importance of your priorities.

Nothing is as good as it seems beforehand.

Wait not if unprepared, but prepare.

Sharpen your axe before chopping down a tree.

A good beginning makes a good ending.

If not confident; check twice.

The mouse that has prepared only one hole
is quickly taken.

Find out what preparation your goal requires.

Apply all your mindmodes to your preparation.

Analyse your potential resources.

An error no wider than a hair
will lead you a hundred miles away from your goal.

Look before you leap,
because snakes creep among sweet flowers.

The aim of preparation
is to manoeuvre yourself in a superior position.

First things first.

Your future depends on what you do right now.

Hope for the best, but prepare for the worst.

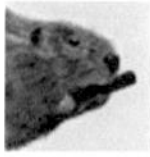

Coming events cast their shadows before them.

Any plan has to be adjusted
to the forever changing reality.

When you prepare, focus on your preparation.

Rain does not stay in the sky.

In handling their affairs,
people fail often close to their success.
Therefore, be as careful at the end
as at the beginning.
Then affairs will not fail [1] §64.

If you've seeded before a heavy rain,
one out of one hundred of your plants will be out of line,
but if you wait and seed later,
only one out of one hundred will take.

The way to hell is paved with good intentions.

Those who could foresee affairs
three days in advance
would be rich for thousands of years.

Do not cut the branch you are sitting on.

Determine what is urgent and what is important.

Prioritize your tasks.

It is no use waiting for your ship to come in,
unless, you have sent one out.

You do not get rice if you plant grass.

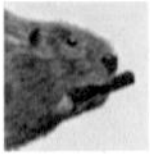

The best preparation for life is nemonik thinking.

Learn to walk before you leap.

Organize your support network.

Do not put the cart before the horse.

Preparation without wisdom
is counterproductive.

Accept

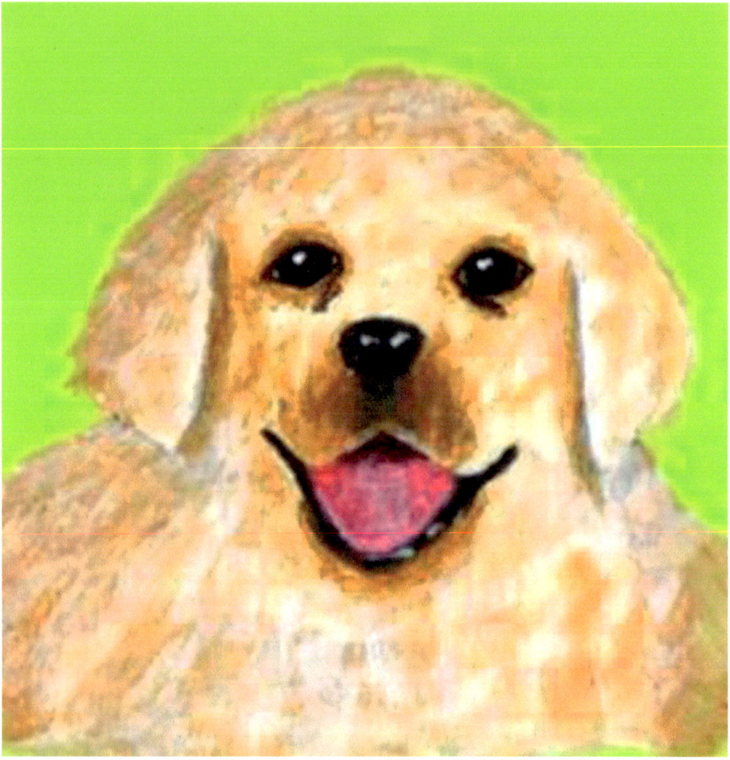

Mantra: I check before I accept.

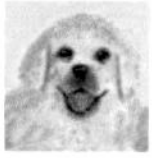

Description Accept

Accept is the nemonik that prompts your mind to accept the incoming information as a true description of the external reality.

True words are not pleasing. Pleasing words are not true [1] §81. True words seem to be paradoxical [1] §78. If you accept all information then you will acquire all true information. However, if your decision-criterion is too lax then you will accept too much false information. Maintain the balance, because it all depends on the situation.

Strength—accepting fosters the acquisition of true information.

Weakness—accepting fosters the acquisition of false information.

Opportunity—accepting could foster the trust of others.

Threat—accepting could foster gullibility, superstition, and shows a lack of logic, wisdom, and common sense. Other people could try to manipulate you with false information or fake news.

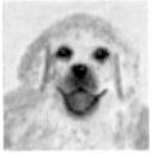

Wisdom relevant to Accept

Accept what you cannot change.

Foster serenity
to accept the things you cannot change.

A vacant mind accepts all suggestions as an empty cave.

Sages accept the search for truth
and reject the urge to win arguments.

Slips of the tongue reveal the truth.

Accept your past in order to improve your future.

Sages accept positioning and reject effort.

Seeing is believing and believing is accepting.

What soberness conceals; drunkenness reveals.

Sages accept compassion and reject rational detachment.

Sages accept justice and reject justifications.

Sages will rule for the stomach and not for the eyes.
Therefore, reject that and accept this [1] §12.

Sages accept dynamic thinking and reject static thinking.

Advice is least heeded when most needed.

Agree between yourselves and I will make it rain.

Do not kill the messenger bringing unwanted tidings.

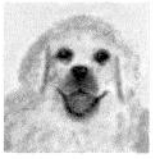

Superior propriety acts
and if there is no agreement,
then the arms are bared [1] §38.

Sages adhere to orthodox agreements
and do not obligate other people by purpose.
Therefore, those with virtue
will uphold the agreement.
Those without virtue
will uphold the details [1] §79.

Sages accept rational thinking and reject rationalizations.

Agree to disagree.

If you do not like it, then you may have to lump it.

If you seek a reputation for wisdom, agree with everyone.

If the cap fits, wear it.

The truth is simple, because it confirms reality.

Do not contradict people just because they contradict you.

There is many a slip between the cup and the lip.

Sages know themselves,
but do not display themselves.
They love themselves,
but do not admire themselves.
Therefore, reject that and accept this [1] §72.

Accept to adjust your goal
if strong balancing forces oppose you.

Sages accept the truth if it cannot be proven wrong.

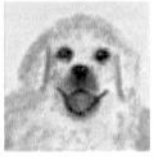

Accept the pressure to act,
in order to act at the right moment.

You cannot judge a book by its cover.

Accept that others joke about you,
but do not joke about others.

Forewarned is forearmed.

Sages accept to achieve success with minimal resources.

Accept everything
and you accept too much misinformation.

Sages accept that all imbalances will be restored
by either artificial or natural forces.

Second thoughts are best.

Sages accept the search for vital questions
and reject pre-set ones.

Sages accept the objective truth
even if it causes emotional pain.

Finding the truth
is more important than winning an argument.

Sages accept
that effort is a signal of inefficiency.

Accept the failures of others, as you accept ugly faces.

Sages accept
that accumulation will evoke balancing forces.

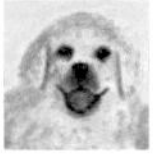

Accept your intuition or you will reject your hidden genius.

Imitation is the sincerest form of flattery.

Children and fools tell the truth.

Accept the country's shame
and be called the Kingdom's leader.
Accept the country's misfortune
and be called the world's King [1] §78.

Accept the unchangeable and change the changeable.

Accept things only after you have considered
to reject them.

Go abroad to hear the truth about home.

There is no acceptance without risk.

Grief for the painful truth, but accept the painful facts.

There is truth in wine.

The truth is seldom spoken.

Few things are seen for ourselves.

If there is smoke, then there is fire.

Admission by the defendant is worth a hundred witnesses.

The unwanted message might be true.

When children stand quiet, they have done some ill.

Reward clear and honest answers.

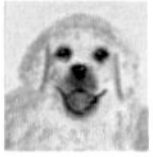

The sting of reproach is in the truth.

Accept that your hidden genius will never explain itself

Sages accept that the restoring force of nature
cannot be opposed by humans.

No answer is an answer.

Accept proactivity
to stop problems growing out of control.

Sages accept critical thinking and reject criticism.

Great people occupy the thick
and do not occupy the thin.
They occupy the fruit,
but do not occupy the fruitless flowers.
Therefore, reject that and accept this [1] §38.

Accept that you live in your inner subjective reality.

Better accepting the bitter facts, than rejecting the truth.

A person who likes eggs, must accept the cackling of hens.

Accept that your reactive mindmode
is superior to all other mindmodes.

To maximize your success,
accept your intuition,
because it is the result of all available information.

Never judge by appearances.

What you see is what you get.

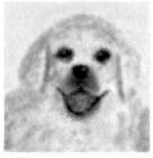

Accept the unpleasing truth, rather than a pleasing lie.

Many truths are spoken in jest.

The truth is stranger than fiction.

Accept the twenty-one nemoniks as tools
that maximize your success.

Great minds think alike.

Accept that one wrong will bring on another.

**Accepting without wisdom
is counterproductive.**

Reject

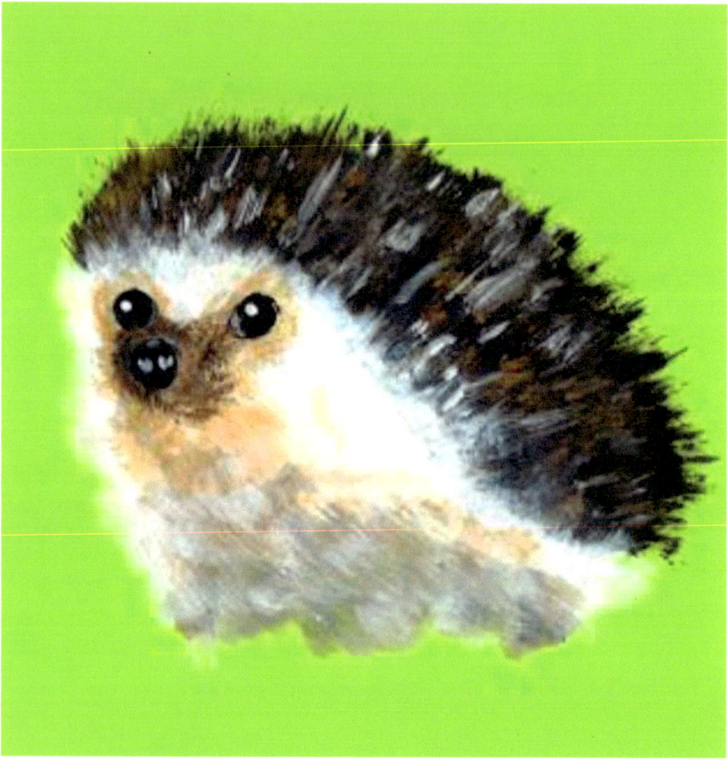

Mantra: I check before I reject.

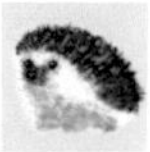

Description Reject

Reject is the nemonik that prompts your mind to reject the incoming information as a true description of the external reality.

Discard adoration and reject artificial knowledge and the people will benefit a hundred times [1] §19. However, if your decision-criterion is too strict then you will also reject too much true information. Maintain the balance, because it all depends on the situation.

Strength—rejecting inhibits the acquisition of false information.

Weakness—rejecting inhibits the acquisition of true information.

Opportunity—rejecting could foster realism, if false information would be rejected. It might prevent traps and ambushes.

Threat—rejecting could foster a high level of criticism of others that it inhibits the support of potential allies.

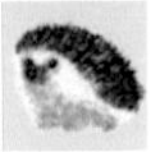

Wisdom relevant to Reject

Those who have motive, opportunity, and means
might bring false messages.

You cannot say yes to everyone.

Sages do not answer vague questions.

Reject things only after you have considered
to accept them.

Accept nothing what you hear,
and only half of what you see.

When in doubt, seek expert advice.

Fire and flax do not agree.

Too good
is too bad.

Complainers
have no need.

There is no currency that buys loyalty.

To hear a Prince's burden is a threat,
rather than an opportunity.

Better safe than sorry.

Some lethal threats
are too small to see.

Silent waters run deep.

If you see a lion,
look for the snake in the grass.

If people deceive me once, shame on them.
If they deceive me twice, shame on me.

Show me a person who never lies
and I will show you a liar.

All that glitters is not gold.

Science is not a democracy.

An idea is not rigth just because it is yours.
An idea is not wrong just because it is not yours.

It is not true just because everyone says so.

A fool never does what a prudent person predicts.

Those who make easy promises are difficult to trust.

There is no greater mistake, then defending a mistake.

Reject gossip, because it needs no carriage.

Appearance is meant to be deceptive.

Hypocrisy is a homage that vice pays to virtue.

Please your eye and hurt your heart.

Rely on your heart to reject lies.

Fools accept only advice that confirms their beliefs.

Sages do not make a mountain out of a molehill.

Things pass for what they seem, rather than what they are.

Beware of the hidden snare.

What people do with you
they will do against you.

The truth is never wrong.

Do not take people's dwellings by force.
Do not reject them a place to live.
Only, if they are not rejected,
they will not reject you [1] §72.

Soften the blow,
because total rejection destroys useful dependency.

The heart never lies,
but is often wrong.

If the great Way is rejected,
then there will be benevolence and justice.
Knowledge and cleverness will appear
and then there is great hypocrisy.
Family relationships will be disharmonious
and then there is animal dirt everywhere.
The State's household will be a confused disorder
and then there is bureaucracy [1] §18.

From the sublime to the ridiculous is a small step.

Situations might be beyond your control,
but your feelings should be under your control.

Snakes prefer to hide under flowers.

The cowl does not make the monk.

Those who are the least, think themselves the most.

A person who gives fair words,
feeds you with an empty spoon.

Fools replace objective thinking with authority.

Empty vessels make the loudest noise.

Watch their emotions, rather than their rhetoric.

A fool tries to give counsel to the wise.

Sages reject extremes,
reject grandeur,
and reject extravagance [1] §29.

Reject in case of doubt.

Sages save people always competently
by not rejecting them.
Not rejected things are resources [1] §27.

Flattery is the velvet that hides the dagger.

A high reward comes with an even higher price.

Fools are those who look like fools
and half of those who do not.

A deer escapes the noise of the drivers,
only to get killed by the waiting hunter.

If words change your emotions,
then someone is pushing your buttons.

It is easy to be wise afterwards.

A flow of words is no proof of being easy.

Discard adoration and reject knowledge
and the people will benefit a hundred times.
Discard benevolence and reject righteousness
and the people will return to filial piety and compassion.
Discard cleverness and reject profit
and there will be no burglars and thieves [1] §19.

Sages are more careful with a person who praises,
than one that criticizes.

True words are not pleasing.
Pleasing words are not true [1] §81.

Success makes even a fool seems wise.

Beware of people
who put your interests before their own.

Elaborate rhetoric conceals the truth.

Galloping and hunting in the field
will madden people's minds.
Goods that are difficult to obtain will harm people.
Therefore, sages will rule for the stomach
and not for the eyes.
Therefore, reject that and accept this [1] §12.

It is better to refuse, than to accept and not to go.

Do not let emotions affect your logic.

Only a great lure works as a lure.

The pot calls the kettle black.

A lure is only a lure if it corrupts prudent judgement.

Only a fool does not recognize a fool.

Who chatters to you will chatter about you.

Manipulators replace objective thinking with rhetoric.

Mice only step in death traps, because of the cheese.

There are many insects around a flowering tree.

Nothing is enough to sell your inner Self.

Do not believe or love too quickly.

Sages reject pre-set questions
and accept the search for vital questions.

Hindsight is always twenty-twenty.

Reject everything
and you reject too much true information.

A person who denies all, confesses all.

The grass is always greener at the other side.

A person who accepts favours, pawns his freedom.

Look for defects, even when it looks right.

Sages care more about substance than novelty.

Do not reject what is popular.

Those promising everything, promise nothing.

The more is promised the less is paid.

Submission to one wrong brings on another.

An angler's bait is designed to look attractive to a fish.

People will tell you lies when you reject the truth.

True emotions do not lie.

Coincidence is often hidden planning.

Do not let emotions cloud your judgement.

A high reward is seldom paid.

One must draw the line somewhere.

Reject empty buzzwords.

Reject noise that is masquerading as reason and logic.

The Venus trap is a deadly heaven for flies.

Reject all you hear and half of what you see.

Reject whims tempting prudence.

Those who make rash promises
are certainly difficult to trust [1] §26.

Barking dogs seldom bite.

Talk is cheap.

Promising shortcuts are often hazardous ambushes.

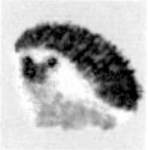

Sages reject criticism and accept critical thinking.

Reject deviations from your questions.

Make sure that you can pay the price in the worst case.

Youth and age will never agree.

Ignore the things that happen between other people.

Sages condemn flattery, rather than rewarding it.

Sages reject winning arguments
and accept the search for truth.

Survival is more important than a huge advance.

Fools ask questions that sages cannot answer.

Reject to risk all.

Rhetoric is the enemy of clarity.

If it is too good to be true, then it most probably is.

Flattery is more destructive than hate,
because it maintains your flaws.

If many were interested, then the reward would be low.

Sages reject detachment and accept compassion.

Too much politeness conceals deceit.

Still waters run deep.

Lies are complex, because they oppose reality.

Sages reject static thinking and accept dynamic thinking.

If it is worth signing,
then it is worth seeking expert advice.

Reject black-box-logic.

Do not say amen to an unacceptable prayer.

Success has many fathers, while failure is an orphan.

Deceit is in a hurry, but honesty can wait at leisure.

Discard knowledge
and there are no worries [1] §19.

They brag most, who can do least.

Sages reject justifications and accept justice.

Opponents might ambush you,
but only friends can betray you.

Eavesdroppers never hear anything
good about themselves.

Dogs do not bark only at thieves.

There is no free lunch.

Fine words butter no parsnip.

Quick and well do not agree.

The greater the reward the greater the risk.

There are two sides to every issue.

It is easier to dam a river, than to stop the flow of gossip.

Sugar is a better bait than vinegar.

Sages reject dogmas and accept dynamic thinking.

Sages know themselves,
but do not display themselves.
They love themselves,
but do not admire themselves.
Therefore, reject that and accept this [1] §72.

Too good, conceals too bad.

Do not let the past distort the present or the future.

Accept that a mountain has moved
before you accept
that people have changed their characters.

Promises are made to be broken.

Despise unsuccessful merit.

Watch out for a very trilling or lame reason
given for something wrong.

No matter how good,
in reality there is always a higher price to be paid.

No one will try to lure you with a rotten egg.

Full of courtesy, full of craft.

The bait hides the hook.

Glittering will blind many fools.

If you want to know the truth,
wait till the argument starts.

Half the truth is a whole lie.

Words are like feathers that are carried off by the wind.

Let others not draw you out to learn your intentions.

A bad payer has always a good excuse.

Praise without profit puts little in the pot.

Sages reject rationalizations
and accept rational thinking.

**Rejecting without wisdom
is counterproductive.**

Reveal

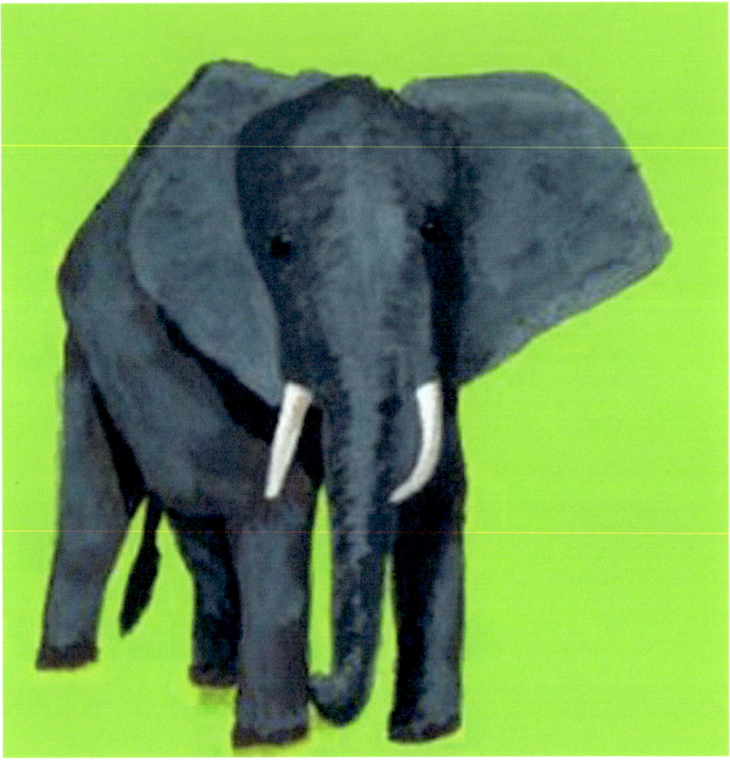

Mantra: I reveal to allies.

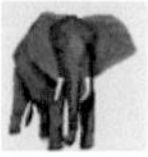

Description Reveal

Reveal is the nemonik that prompts your mind to project true information to the external reality.

Sages carry out their teachings without rhetoric [1] §2. Competent people are the teachers of incompetent people [1] §27. The teachers of humanity discus and teach people that violent people will achieve nothing but death [1] §42. Sages are always without opinions. They use the opinions of common people as their opinions [1] §49.

Strength—revealing fosters simplicity, because you have little to hide. It is hard to remember deceptions correctly and fit them continuously into the changing reality. The truth is easy to remember.

Weakness—revealing fosters your predictability, because other people know your intentions and plans.

Opportunity—revealing could gain trust, because you would be perceived as reliable and honest.

Threat—revealing could get you trapped and ambushed by your opponents, because they can predict you.

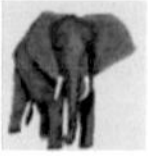

Wisdom relevant to Reveal

There is no revelation without risk.

A liar is not believed when he tells the truth.

Showing disbelief makes fools spit out their secrets.

Make yourself all honey and the flies will devour you.

Brevity is the soul of wit.

A bad excuse is better than none.

Sages apply critical thinking to foster the truth,
rather than criticism to win the argument.

Showing respect is the basis for friendship.

Fake it, if you cannot make it.

Cry wolf too often and no help will come anymore.

Make sure that your first impressions are lasting.

Who stays quiet agrees.

A polite devil is more acceptable than a rude saint.

Break your word and you break your credibility.

Avoid contradicting others
and others will not contradict you.

Always talk about others
as if they were standing next to you.

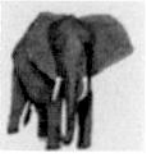

Do not make yourself a mouse, or the cat will eat you.

Sages apply justice to foster the truth,
rather than justifications to win the argument.

Be careful with promises,
because reality will never match the imagination of others.

Feigned doubt is the master key to the secrets of fools.

Success never needs an excuse.

The word of honest people is their bond.

Words that come from the heart
stay warm three winters long.

Arrogance causes ignorance.

A fault confessed is half redressed.

To break a promise is worse than refusing a request.

Speak sparsely.

One picture is worth ten thousand words.

Do as I say, not as I do.

Showing is believing.

Bestow favours yourself.
Let others refuse requests.

Resemble a King in excellence.

Confession is good for the soul.

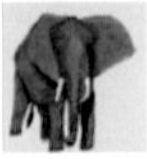

Any publicity is good publicity.

Sages reveal things only after they have considered
to conceal them.

Reveal your talents only at the right time and place.

A soft word turns away fury.

A person who gets a name for early rising
can stay in bed until midday.

There is nothing that costs less than civility.

Showing off talent may backfire.

There is not such a thing as bad publicity.

Repay hatred with kindness [1] §63.

Do not halloo until you are out of the woods.

Better to ask a question than to remain ignorant.

Know how to use subtle insinuation.

Honesty is the best policy.

Stick to the truth,
because a liar needs a good memory.

Speak well of the dead.

Silence means consent.

Self-praise ruins your reputation.

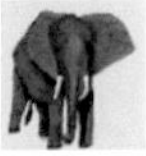

Show modesty and embrace simplicity [1] §19.

Winning an argument does not mean that
you have convinced your opponent.

A lure is never too good to be a lure.

The tailor makes the person.

Sages carry out their teachings without speaking [1] §2.

One can forgive a murder but not impoliteness.

Good wine needs no label.

A civil question deserves a civil answer.

The one who digs deepest gets muddiest.

A silly question deserves a silly answer.

Express yourself earnestly
and you have no reason for shame
even if you lack talent.

You cannot be a howling success by simply howling.

The frowning face of a goat
does not prevent it being slaughtered.

Speak what needs to be said, or stay silent.

Either remain quiet,
or say things that improve the silence.

Speak fair and think what you like.

Competent speakers pursue no flaws [1] §27.

Remain interesting and have many topics for discussions.

Flies are attracted by sugar, rather than vinegar.

Examples are better than commands.

Spend words as efficiently as money.

Those who talk much say little.
Those who talk little say much.

It is good enough to convince the wise.

Persuade without words.

One deceit evokes the need for many others.

A person who has no silver in his purse
should have silk in his tongue.

Trouble shared is trouble halved.

Almost and about are words that prevent lying.

If you know little,
stick to what is tried and tested.

Hide your light not under a bushel.

Add courtesy to what you sell.

Sages are always without opinions.
They use the opinions of common people
as their opinions [1] §49.

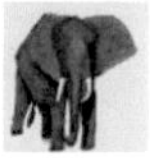

Old people may miss their target with a stone,
but never with their word.

A problem shared is a problem halved.

Love, grief, and money cannot be concealed.

Call a spade a spade.

If you do not know, then ask an expert.

Painful jokes are never agreeable.

Be unpredictable; alternate guile with innocence.

Teaching without speaking and Non-action
will benefit the whole world [1] §43.

Ask questions, because there is no shame in ignorance.

A good tale is none the worse for being told twice.

A lie can take you far away, but without hope of return.

Fling enough dirt and some will stick.

Deceit always returns on its creator.

A person who asks a question is a fool for a minute;
he who does not ask a question remains a fool forever.

What is invisible might as well not exist.

Stop rumours at the source.

Special things are devaluated by praising common things.

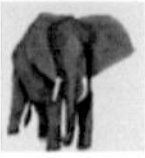

Avoid to say no, by changing the topic.

The pen is mightier than the sword.

A person who prides himself on his ancestry
is like the potato plant;
the best part of which is underground.

A word to the wise is enough.

I am valuable to those few who understand me.
Therefore, sages wear cheap cloth
that conceals jade [1] §70.

Give credit where credit is due.

Be straightforward in all your dealings
and noble with strangers.

One who shouts obtains more than ten who remain silent.

There is a time to speak and a time to be silent.

The squeaking wheel gets the oil.

Give a lie a twenty-four hours start,
and you can never overtake it.

Anyone can be polite to a king,
but it takes a sage to be polite to a beggar.

Clothes make the person.

Humour is a better teacher than seriousness.

Say something nice or say nothing at all.

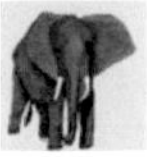

Fling enough dirt and some will stick on you.

Those of value speak about their plans
and succeed in completing their affairs.
Yet, the common people will say;
it happened naturally [1] §17.

Make sure to bark up the right tree.

Practice what you preach.

Words cut deeper than swords.

Courtesy costs nothing.

Force may lead to agreement,
but only the truth will lead to conviction.

Better to ask the way than go astray.

Sages apply rational thinking to foster the truth,
rather than rationalizations to win the argument.

The word that remains in the belly
does not mean anything.

It is better to refuse
than to break a promise.

A liar needs a good memory.

You break your word once
and you break your name forever.

In speaking, the goodness is truth [1] §8.

Your word is your bond.

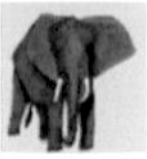

Laugh and the world laughs with you,
weep and you weep alone.

A broken promise
will hunt you forever.

Speak only after you have thought.

Evil communications corrupt good manners.

First impressions are most lasting.

Imitation is the sincerest form of flattery.

Praise the favours done to you,
because that motivates others to do more for you.

Revealing without wisdom
is counterproductive.

Conceal

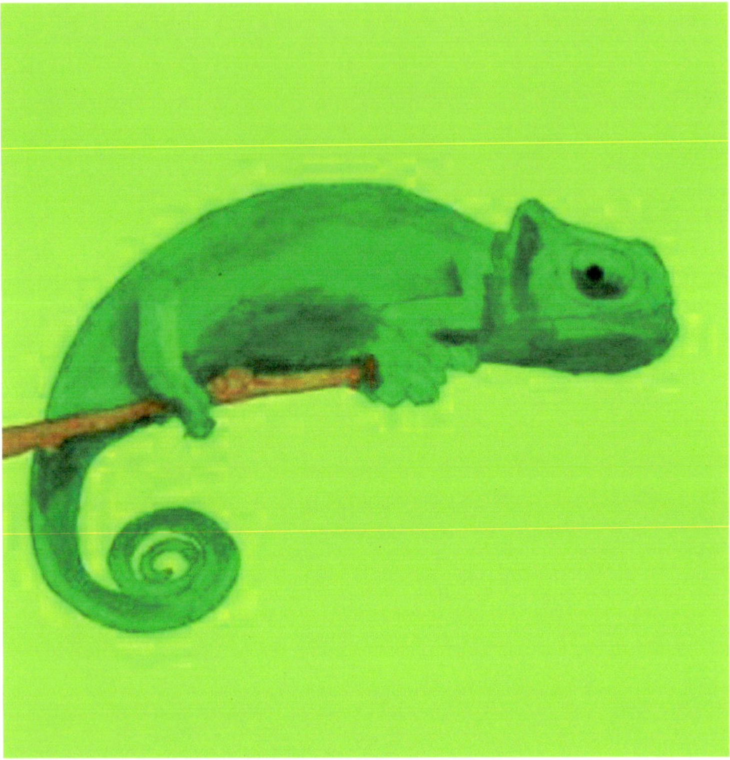

Mantra: I conceal from opponents.

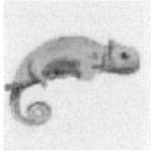

Description Conceal

Conceal is the nemonik that prompts your mind to hide true information from the external reality.

Sages wear cheap cloth that conceals jade [1] §70. Stop the gossip and close the doors; and to the end of life there will be no hard work. Start the gossip and meddle in affairs; and to the end of life there will be no safety [1] §52. Sages who desire to be above the people must place themselves below them [1] §66.

Strength—concealing makes you unpredictable and therefore hard to ambush.

Weakness—concealing fosters complexity, because it is hard to remember deceptions correctly and adjust them continuously to the changing reality. The truth is easier to remember.

Opportunity—concealing could foster the possibility to trap and ambush opponents.

Threat—concealing could foster distrust, because you might be perceived as unreliable and dishonest.

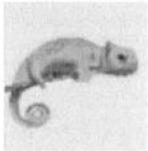

Wisdom relevant to Conceal

Camouflage is the first line of defence.

Those who hide, know best how to find.

A closed mouth catches no flies.

Maintain your superiority by holding back.

The arrow that has left the bow never returns.

Memory fades, letters remain.

Hush until you heal.

A paper wrapping cannot conceal a fire.

Keep others guessing the depths of your talents.

Better to be thought a fool,
than to open your mouth and remove all doubt.

Think before you speak.

Do not quarrel with your bread and butter.

A sage has much to say and yet remains silent.

Words fly, writings remain.

Do not wash your dirty linen in public.

Never tell an evil person about your misfortune.

Revealing your ultimate goal may backfire.

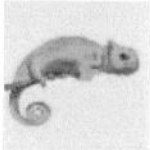

Who asks at once for a lot,
returns home with an empty bag.

Little cups have large ears.

Once a traitor, always a traitor.

In vain, the net is spread within sight of the bird.

Sages do not desire to display their knowledge [1] §77.

Keep your cards to your chest.

If you cannot bite, then never show your teeth.

A defence in writing leaves a trail against you.

A traitor has no country.

Confess and be hanged.

Pouring oil on the fire is not the way to quench it.

Do not sell your soul.
You have to live with it.

A person who keeps a secret prevents much mischief.

Do not whirl a killed snake in the air,
because the remaining ones will see you.

Carefully conceal what shows a small heart.

Write your intentions in code.

Never tell your enemy that your foot aches.

Treason is loved, but traitors are hated.

A word spoken is past recalling.

One written word stays longer than hundred spoken.

Never make threats you cannot carry out.

You show your cards and you risk losing the game.

A bleating sheep loses a bite.

A still tongue makes a wise head.

Do not show your hand if you want to win the card game.

When the heart overflows,
it comes out through the mouth.

Never ask pardon before you are accused.

A secret remains a secret only when one person knows it.

We must have reasons for speech,
but we need none for silence.

Silence gives consent.

Two may keep a secret if one of them is dead.

All cats are grey in the dark.

Don't cry before you are hurt.

Do not explain to those who do not ask for it.

Bringing bad news without remedy may backfire.

Prudency shuns luminance.

Behave as if others are watching.

People might value gossip,
but the wise will never thrust the bringer
with a secret.

Better to beg forgiveness, than to ask permission.

Silence can be more revealing than words.

Do not explain your ideas clearly
if complexity is more valued.

An ounce of discretion is worth a pound of wit.

Walls have ears.

Call attention to yourself
and your talents will be turned into defects.

Sages do not boast about themselves.
Therefore, they have merit [1] §22.

Do not teach your grandmother to suck eggs.

Do not take your harp to the party.

Those who know do not speak.
Those who speak do not know [1] §56.

It is a foolish sheep that makes the wolf his confessor.

Sages do not display themselves.
Therefore, they are brilliant [1] §22.

Not all truth should be spoken.

Conceal things only after you have considered
to reveal them.

Pretend it is not you who rejects.

Words are like arrows, they cannot be withdrawn.

Self-praise is no recommendation.

Do not tell tales out of school.

Those living in glasshouses should not throw stones.

When all people speak, no one listens.

Reason not with the great, it is a perilous gate.

Good wine needs no advertising.

Do not talk the talk, if you cannot walk the walk.

The tongue ever turns to the aching tooth.

Exaggeration shows a lack of knowledge and prudence.

An arrow can be pulled out of a wound,
but a hurtful word stays forever in the heart.

You can catch more flies with honey than vinegar.

Few drink and remain wise; most lose all their senses.

Those who talk much say little.
Those who talk little say much.

The truth is often used as a weapon of destruction.

When the word is out, it belongs to someone else.

It is no good harping on a frayed string.

There's plenty of time to bemoan bad fortune
once it arrives.

Let people have weapons
without displaying them [1] §80.

Do not trust your honour to others
without having theirs in return.

If you do not have anything nice to say,
do not say anything at all.

Do not invite approval or flattery from others.

A word and a stone once thrown away
cannot be returned.

Loose lips sink ships.

A fish should not leave the deep water [1] §36.

If you do not know, smile and look wise (Sijbrand).

Curses are like chickens, they come home to roost.

A silent fool appears to be wise.

Silence is the hallmark of the wise.

Alcohol will preserve anything but a secret.

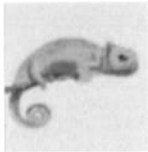

People who excuse themselves
before being accused,
accuse themselves.

If you cannot wear the skin of a lion,
then weir the skin of a fox.

Those who display themselves
are without brilliance.
Those who regard themselves
are without honour.
Those who boast about themselves
are without merit.
Those who are arrogant
are without development [1] §24.

A person who takes responsibility becomes a public target.

Least said, soonest mended.

I am valuable to those few who understand me.
Therefore, sages wear cheap cloth
that conceals jade [1] §70.

Noble deeds are done in silence.

A bird set free may return,
but a word escaping your lips will not.

Discretion is the better part of valour.

Light not a candle to the sun.

Talking repeats only what you know already.

The tongue is not steel, yet it cuts deep.

If you do not want to hear lies,
then do not ask questions.

When the hunter returns
and is carrying mushrooms,
do not ask him about his hunt.

Three in ten people live extremely
and move into the realm of death.
What is the reason?
That is because they live extremely.
They are incompetent in hiding, listening,
and conserving their lives [1] §50.

Speaking seldom is natural,
because strong storms
do not drum all morning [1] §23.

One lie makes many.

Do not talk about yourself,
because it reveals either vainness or meekness.

Have a cough and your smoking will not remain secret.

Keep your audience in suspense.

Fools are like all other people
as long as they remain silent.

Speak not of the debts of others
unless you pay for them.

Hide your hidden agenda.

A blindside requires blinded people.

A person cannot speak well
who cannot hold his tongue.

Fools do not know how to conceal their foolishness.

To mock your elders
is to wreck the house
where you have to stay tonight.

There is always time to speak
and never time to take it back.

Never complain,
because that justifies others to do the same to you.

Proclamations will be criticized.

It is dangerous to share secrets
with those greater than you.

A person who excuses himself accuses himself.

Conceal your weakness,
because malice will focus on it.

Silence is golden.

The truth can do inhumane damage beyond repair.

Sages know themselves,
but do not display themselves [1] §72.

Fools are eloquent when they stay silent.

Listening, rather than speaking provides information.

A silent person is never wrong.

Princes should not be given bitter cures.

See no evil, hear no evil, speak no evil.

Speaking is silver, but silence is gold.

Concealing without wisdom is counterproductive.

SUMMARY

This manual provides the wisdom for Nemonik Thinking in the form of proverbs. An exhaustive network of 21 keywords, called nemoniks, prompts the mind to associate each memorized nemonik with the relevant proverbs in order to make better decisions. Rather than providing clear cut solutions; each proverb prompts the mind to think and evaluate the value of the proverb for the particular situation. Hence, some proverbs might be relative to more than one nemonik or even opposite nemoniks. Nemonik Thinking is an extension of Lao Zi's *Dao De Jing* [5, 6, 7, 8, 1] and explained in my other books [2, 3, 9, 10, 4, 11, 12].

APPENDICES

Glossary

ACCEPT—nemonik that prompts the mind to maximize success by accepting the incoming information as a true description of the reality.

ACCUMULATE—nemonik that prompts the mind to maximize success by increasing the amount of matter that is under control.

ACT—nemonik that prompts the mind to maximize success by changing or moving matter in space and time.

ADVANCE—nemonik that prompts the mind to maximize success by decreasing the distance to the goal.

Affecter—mental signal generated by a subconscious mindset that influences the conscious.

Affectorial Thinking—subconscious way of Dynamic Thinking that creates mindsets. Affectorial Thinking includes the Creative and Reactive mindmodes. See Rational Thinking.

Association—See Free-association and Guided-association.

BALANCE—nemonik that prompts the mind to maximize success by maintaining the Yin-Yang balances, which prevents counterproductive rebalances.

Brainware—set of material components comprising the Central Nerve System. See Mindware.

Cognitive dissonance—individual rejection of correct information in order to protect incorrect subconscious information by evoking individual stress, fear, frustration, anger, aggression, etc. See Groupthink.

Cognitive procedures—include memory and thinking.

Collective-mindmode—specific way of Rational-thinking that applies rhetoric in order to reach social agreements that are compiled in the temporary rules of people.

COLLECTIVE—nemonik that prompts the conscious mind to maximize success by using Rational Thinking in order to deal with people.

CONCEAL—nemonik that prompts the mind to maximize success by hiding true information from the reality.

Concentrated-Relaxation—tool of Mind Management that evokes semiconscious dominance by reducing conscious-dominance without falling asleep. It includes: muscle and breathing awareness; evoking semiconscious dominance; progressive muscle relaxation and breathing; deepening semiconscious; creating mindsets with mantras; returning conscious dominance; and mind-slide.

Conscious dominance—healthy mental state of being awake that is mutually exclusive from subconscious dominance and is fostered by concentration. See Mind.

Conscious—relatively small part of the mind that is dominant when awake; aware of the reality and the Self; manages the mind; and maximizes success with Rational Thinking. See Mind.

Conventional Thinking—educational competitive-memory based way of conscious thinking that aims to win competitions in the external reality by using free-association. Conventional Thinking fosters systemic cognitive failure and manmade extinction problems. See Nemonik Thinking.

Creative-mindmode—specific way of Affectorial-thinking that deals with the future and unique problems by hypothetically randomizing available information in order to create new information such as: ideas, innovations, and intuitions.

CREATIVE—nemonik that prompts the subconscious mind to maximize success by using Affectorial Thinking in order to deal with unique problems.

DISPOSE—nemonik that prompts the mind to maximize success by decreasing the amount of matter that is under control.

Dynamic Thinking—part of Nemonik Thinking that maximizes external success by using 21 nemoniks to adjust that way of thinking to the situation. Dynamic Thinking includes Rational and Affectorial Thinking. Dynamic Thinking fosters productive freedom, harmony, win-win strategies, cooperation, and unification. See Static and Nemonik Thinking.

Educational thinking—See Conventional thinking.

EFFICIENT—nemonik that prompts the mind to maximize success with a minimum of effort and resources by aligning with restoring forces.

External reality—surrounds your mind and includes space, matter, and time. See Reality.

Firewall—subconscious cognitive tool that protects the genius from external and internal interference and manifests itself as cognitive dissonance and groupthink.

FOCUS—nemonik that prompts the mind to concentrate on maximizing success. Success is to obtain what you seek and escape what you suffer.

Free-association—cognitive procedure that activates spontaneously a link between two or more pieces of information. See Guided-association.

Genius—part of the subconscious that prevent a conscious information-overload by storing and processing that information and executing all inherited and learned skills.

Groupthink—collective rejection of correct information in order to protect incorrect collective information by evoking collective stress, fear, frustration, anger, aggression, etc. See Cognitive Dissonance.

Guided-association—cognitive procedure that activates a memorized link between a nemonik and the icon, definition, potential questions, SWOT-analyses, mantras, and proverbs for that nemonik. See Free-association.

Hegel, George Wilhelm Frederich (1770-1831) —German philosopher who introduced Hegel's dialectic describing the progress of knowledge.

Hegel's dialectic—during the first stage of this dialectic, a tested description of reality is introduced that is called the thesis. During the second stage, that thesis is challenged by a tested and conflicting description of reality that is called the antithesis. During the third stage, this conflict is resolved by merging the thesis and antithesis in a synthesis. The synthesis becomes the new thesis and the process repeats itself. Consequently, the development of knowledge is a process and, therefore, knowledge is temporary.

Humphrey, Albert, S. (1926-2005) —introduced the concept of SWOT-analyses.

Ignorance—lack of knowledge.

Internal reality—mental perception of the external reality. See Reality.

Knowledge—valid and reliable description of reality.

Lateral thinking—way of creative thinking that reformulates problems and looks at them from different perspectives in order to generate ideas and find solutions. Edward de Bono introduced that way of thinking in his book 'Lateral Thinking' (1970).

Manmade Extinction Problems (MEP)—include climate change, nuclear war, dwindling resources, overpopulation, industrial pollution, extinction of species, and the overall destruction of nature that are caused by Conventional Thinking.

Mantra—tool of Mind Management comprising a word or phrase that is repeated consciously during semiconscious dominance in order to manage the subconscious mindsets. See Concentrated-Relaxation.

Memory—cognitive procedure that stores, maintains, and recalls knowledge in order to preserve it across space and time. See Thinking.

Mental Firewall—See Firewall.

Mental state—distinct level of awareness such as conscious dominance, subconscious dominance, semiconscious dominance, and unconsciousness.

Meta-thinking—thinking about thinking.

Mind Management—part of Nemonik Thinking that maximizes internal success by using Concentrated-Relaxation and Mantras. The aim of Mind Management is fostering conscious management of the subconscious genius by opening their semiconscious communication channel. See Nemonik Thinking.

Mindmode—special way of thinking that deals with a particular topic. Mindmodes are Objective, Collective, Creative, and Reactive.

Mind—nonmaterial part of a person that includes all conscious, semiconscious, and subconscious processes and structures resulting from interactions between the brainware and mindware of that person. The Mind comprises the Conscious, Semiconscious, and Subconscious.

Mindset—habituated set of rules or algorithms that generates affecters. See Creative and Reactive Mindsets.

Mindware—set of rules or algorithms that tells the brainware how to create and maintain the mind. Mindware could be compared to the software of a computer.

Mnemonic—cognitive tool that activates the memory. See Nemonik.

Nemonik Accelerator—cognitive tool that increases the speed of your thinking by fostering agreement during disagreement, while fostering disagreement during agreement. The nemonik-accelerator is based on Hegel's dialectic.

Nemonik Associative Network (NAN)—subconscious construction linking an exhaustive set of 21 keywords called nemoniks with guided-association to an almost infinite amount of well-organized problem-solving tools.

Nemonik Thinking—conscious, semiconscious, and subconscious way of thinking that maximizes external success with Dynamic Thinking and internal success with Mind Management.

Nemonik—memorized keyword that recalls associated problem-solving information from memory and activates the processing of information in order to create new information. The 21 nemoniks are: Focus, Balance, Efficient, Proactive; Objective, Collective, Creative, Reactive; Advance, Stay, Retreat; Accumulate, Preserve, Dispose; Act, Wait, Prepare, Accept, Reject, Reveal, and Conceal. See Mnemonic.

Objective-mindmode—specific way of Rational-thinking that applies logic in order to discover the true and immutable laws of nature.

OBJECTIVE—nemonik that prompts the conscious mind to maximize success by using Rational Thinking in order to deal with nature.

PREPARE—nemonik that prompts the mind to maximize success by getting ready for the most productive action.

PRESERVE—nemonik that prompts the mind to maximize success by maintaining the same amount of matter that is under control.

PROACTIVE—nemonik that prompts the mind to maximize success by restoring the balance before the problem grows.

Problem—anything that inhibits the maximization of your success. Many phenomena only appear to be problems.

Procrastination—counterproductive delay. It is a thief of time and opportunities.

Rational Thinking—conscious way of Dynamic Thinking that submits valid and reliable descriptions of reality to logic in order to create new valid and reliable descriptions of reality. Rational Thinking includes the Objective and Collective mindmodes. See Affectorial Thinking.

Reactive-mindmode—specific way of Affectorial-thinking that utilizes experiences of the past to generate mindsets, which produce affecters such as: skills, habits, and emotions.

REACTIVE—nemonik that prompts the subconscious mind to maximize success by using Affectorial Thinking in order to deal with repetitive problems.

Reality—includes External and Internal realities.

REJECT—nemonik that prompts the mind to maximize success by rejecting the incoming information as a true description of the reality.

RETREAT—nemonik that prompts the mind to maximize success by increasing the distance to the goal.

REVEAL—nemonik that prompts the mind to maximize success by projecting true information to the reality.

Semiconscious dominance—drowsy healthy state of mind between conscious and subconscious dominance that is fostered by Concentrated-Relaxation. Every time you fall asleep or wake-up slowly, you will slide through semiconscious dominance. See Mind.

Semiconscious—part of the mind that manages the communication between the conscious and subconscious with an adjustable firewall. See Mind.

Silent mind—mental state that activates the subconscious without conscious interference, which is often used to cope with emergencies. Also referred to as the Empty Mind or Zone.

Static thinking—part of Conventional Thinking that aims to maximize winning in the external reality by adjusting the situation to a fixed way of thinking. Static thinking fosters counterproductive control, conflict, win-lose strategies, competition, and polarization. See Dynamic Thinking.

STAY—nemonik that prompts the mind to maximize success by maintaining the same distance to the goal.

Subconscious dominance—healthy state of being asleep that is mutually exclusive from conscious dominance and fostered by relaxation. Nevertheless, the subconscious could become dominant during an emergency. See Mind.

Subconscious—largest part of the mind that is dominant when asleep; stores and processes bulk information; consciously inaccessible; and maximizes success with Affectorial Thinking. See Mind.

Success—"obtain what you seek and escape what you suffer" [2] §62.

SWOT-analysis—problem-solving tool that evaluates the Strengths, Weaknesses, Opportunities, and Threats of each nemonik in comparison to the actual situation. Strength is an intrinsic advantage; Weakness is an intrinsic disadvantage; Opportunity is a potential advantage; and Threat is a potential disadvantage. SWOT-analyses were introduced by the American business consultant Albert S. Humphrey (1926-2005).

Systemic Cognitive Failure (SCF)—static thinking in a hyperdynamic reality that has created a triangle of doom. Education fosters science; Science fosters technology; Technology fosters manmade extinction problems. Conventional Thinking fosters systemic cognitive failure. Systemic cognitive failure is maintained by cognitive dissonance and groupthink.

Thinking—cognitive procedure that processes available knowledge in order to generate new knowledge. It includes: affectorial, analytical, collective, creative, critical, dynamic, intuitive-emotive, lateral, left-brain, legalistic, logical, objective, rational, reactive, right-brain, scientific, strategic, static, and systems thinking. See Conventional Thinking and Cognitive procedures.

Triangle of Doom—education fosters science; science fosters technology; technology fosters manmade extinction problems.

Unconscious—unhealthy mental state that is characterized by the absence of mental activity. See Mind.

WAIT—nemonik that prompts the mind to maximize success by delaying action until it is the most productive time for that action.

Winning—defeating others in competition.

Wisdom—productive application of knowledge.

References

[1] Schade, A., Stunning Revelations about Lao Zi's Dao De Jing, 2 ed., Dunedin NZ: nemonik-thinking.org (Printer Amazon), 2017.

[2] Schade, A., Maximum Success with Nemonik Thinking, Dunedin NZ: nemonik-thinking.org (Printer Amazon), 2022.

[3] Schade, A., Survival: A manual for Nemonik Thinking, Dunedin NZ: nemonik-thinking.org (Printer Amazon), 2022.

[4] Schade, A., "Ancient Theory Challenges Modern Physics," in *Maximum Success with Nemonik Thinking - Ancient Wisdom*, Dunedin NZ, nemonik-thinking.org (Printer Amazon), 2021.

[5] Schade, A., Dictionary Lao Zi's Dao De Jing, Dunedin NZ: nemonik-thinking.org (Printer Amazon), 2018.

[6] Schade, A., Meta-translation Lao Zi's Dao De Jing (1-37), 3 ed., vol. 2, Dunedin NZ: nemonik-thinking.org (Printer Amazon), 2018.

[7] Schade, A., Meta-translation Lao Zi's Dao De Jing (38-81), 3 ed., vol. 3, Dunedin NZ: nemonik-thinking.org (Printer Amazon), 2018.

[8] Schade, A., Lao Zi's Dao De Jing Demystified, 2 ed., vol. 4, Dunedin NZ: nemonik-thinking.org (Printer Amazon), 2017.

[9] Schade, A., Knowledge, Dunedin NZ: nemonik-thinking.org (Printer Amazon), 2022 (planned).

[10] Schade, A., Nemonik Information System (NIS), Dunedin NZ: nemonik-thinking.org, 2022.

[11] Schade, A., "Ancient Theory Challenges Modern Psychology," in *Maximum Success with Nemonik Thinking - Ancient Wisdom*, Dunedin NZ, nemonik-thinking.org (Printer Amazon), 2021.

[12] Schade, A., "The Cognitive Revolution," in *Maximum Success with Nemonik Thinking - Ancient Wisdom*, Dunedin NZ, nemonik-thinking.org (Printer Amazon), 2021.

[13] Schade, A., Simplification, Dunedin NZ: nemonik-thinking.org (Printer Amazon), 2022.

[14] Schade, A., Education Kills Humanity, Dunedin NZ: nemonik-thinking.org (Printer Amazon), 2016.

[15] Schade, A., Lao Zi's Dao De Jing Demystified, 2 ed., vol. 4, Dunedin: nemonik-thinking.org (Printer Amazon), 2017, p. 478.

[16] Schade, A., Stunning Revalations about Lao Zi's Dao De Jing, 2 ed., vol. 5, Dunedin NZ: nemonik-thinking.org (Printer Amazon), 2017.

List of Figures

My Other Books

Dictionary Lao Zi's Dao De Jing [5]

This Chinese-English and English-Chinese dictionary is especially compiled for the translation of Lao Zi's ancient book Dao De Jing (Schade, Meta-translation Lao Zi's Dao De Jing (1-37), 2018) and (Schade, Meta-translation Lao Zi's Dao De Jing (38-81), 2018). Dao De Jing means literally—A Classic about the Way of Nature and the Way of People. It aims to maximize your success, which is to obtain what you seek and escape what you suffer. Success is maximized by aligning the Way of People with the Way of Nature (Schade, Stunning Revelations about Lao Zi's Dao De Jing, 2017). The Chinese versions used in this study include— (Wang Bi, 226-249 AD); (He-Shang Gong, 179-157 BC); (Fu Yi, ~200 BC); (Mawangdui (A), ~200 BC); (Mawangdui (B), ~200 BC); and (Guodian, ~300 BC). Together, those versions contain about 1,600 different pictographs. Every language changes over time and, therefore, some of Lao Zi's ancient pictographs are not used anymore, while the meaning of others has changed. In addition, most modern Chinese pictographs have several English meanings that foster ambiguity. Therefore, the exhaustive English meanings for each pictograph were extracted from reputable sources. Furthermore, a system of Digital Index for Pictographs (DIP) is introduced that simplifies the digital classification of Chinese pictographs.

Meta-translation Lao Zi's Dao... (1-37) [6]

The title of Lao Zi's ancient book Dao De Jing means literally—A Classic about the Way of Nature and the Way of People. Dao De Jing aims to maximize your success, which is to obtain what you seek and escape what you suffer. Success is maximized by aligning the Way of People with the Way of Nature (Schade, Stunning Revelations about Lao Zi's Dao De Jing, 2017). Despite the great efforts, previous translations of Dao De Jing do not present an adequate understanding of that mysterious manuscript. In order to take optimal advantage of the expertise accumulated in such earlier studies, this meta-translation is based on an English meta-analysis and a Chinese meta-analysis. The English meta-analysis is based on the following English translations—(Chan Wing-Tsit, 1988); (Cheng Gia-Fu and English, J, 1972); (Henricks, Lao-Tzu: Te-Tao Ching, 1993); (Land, 1990); (Lau, Lao Tzu: Tao Te Ching, 1985); (Lin, J. P., 1977); (Man-ho Kwok; Palmer, M.; & Ramsay, J., 1997); (Waley, 1968); and (Wing, 1986). The Chinese meta-analysis is based on the following Chinese versions of Dao De Jing— (Wang Bi, 226-249 AD); (He-Shang Gong, 179-157 BC); (Fu Yi, ~200 BC); (Mawangdui (A), ~200 BC); (Mawangdui (B), ~200 BC); and (Guodian, ~300 BC). This meta-translation of Dao (Chapters 1-37) is based on a special dictionary (Schade, Dictionary Lao Zi's Dao De Jing, 2018), while it is the foundation for (Schade, Lao Zi's Dao De Jing Demystified, 2017).

Meta-translation Lao Zi's Dao... (38-81) [7]

The title of Lao Zi's ancient book Dao De Jing means literally—A Classic about the Way of Nature and the Way of People. Dao De Jing aims to maximize your success, which is to obtain what you seek and escape what you suffer. Success is maximized by aligning the Way of People with the Way of Nature (Schade, Stunning Revelations about Lao Zi's Dao De Jing, 2017). Despite the great efforts, previous translations of Dao De Jing do not present an adequate understanding of that mysterious manuscript. In order to take optimal advantage of the expertise accumulated in such earlier studies, this meta-translation is based on an English meta-analysis and a Chinese meta-analysis. The English meta-analysis is based on the following English translations—(Chan Wing-Tsit, 1988); (Cheng Gia-Fu and English, J, 1972); (Henricks, Lao-Tzu: Te-Tao Ching, 1993); (Land, 1990); (Lau, Lao Tzu: Tao Te Ching, 1985); (Lin, J. P., 1977); (Man-ho Kwok; Palmer, M.; & Ramsay, J., 1997); (Waley, 1968); and (Wing, 1986). The Chinese meta-analysis is based on the following Chinese versions of Dao De Jing— (Wang Bi, 226-249 AD); (He-Shang Gong, 179-157 BC); (Fu Yi, ~200 BC); (Mawangdui (A), ~200 BC); (Mawangdui (B), ~200 BC); and (Guodian, ~300 BC). This meta-translation of De (Chapters 38-81) is based on a special dictionary (Schade, Dictionary Lao Zi's Dao De Jing, 2018), while it is the foundation for (Schade, Lao Zi's Dao De Jing Demystified, 2017).

Lao Zi's Dao De Jing Demystified [14]

The title of Lao Zi's ancient book Dao De Jing means literally—A Classic about the Way of Nature and the Way of People. It aims to maximize your success, which is to obtain what you seek and escape what you suffer. Success is maximized by aligning the Way of People with the Way of Nature. The current study presents four English versions of increasing demystification. The first one is the Meta-translation version as developed in (Schade, Meta-translation Lao Zi's Dao De Jing (1-37), 2018) and (Schade, Meta-translation Lao Zi's Dao De Jing (38-81), 2018). However, Lao Zi's poetic style, mysticism, metaphors, and synonyms are still inhibiting a clear understanding. The second one is the Clarification version, which is presented in parallel with the Meta-translation. That clarification increased the consistency of Lao Zi's terminology, but significant chapters about Dao are still located in the De section and vice versa. Therefore, the third one is the Chapters Reorganized version in which the chapters are relocated to the Dao and De sections. Nevertheless, the text remains fuzzy, because several chapters relate to both sections. Therefore, the fourth one is the Sentences Reorganized version in which the sentences are sorted by topic. That version is the foundation for (Schade, Stunning Revelations about Lao Zi's Dao De Jing, 2017).

Stunning Revelations about Lao Zi... [15]

The title of Lao Zi's ancient book Dao De Jing means in modern terminology—A Classic about the Physics of Psychology. Dao De Jing is a significant contribution of the Chinese literature to the contemporary sciences of physics and psychology. Lao Zi presents a sophisticated theory concerning the origin, formation, and working of the universe. Although that theory is at the cutting edge of modern physics, it provides a simple and practical principle. That principle holds that the unstoppable force Qi will always maintain the multitude of Yin-Yang balances comprising our universe. Therefore, Lao Zi's theory of psychology predicts that people can only maximize their success by aligning with Qi. Success is to obtain what you seek and escape what you suffer. Unfortunately, humanity has ignored Lao Zi's principles for two-and-halve thousand years. As a result, we are now facing manmade problems such as climate change, continuous warfare, dwindling resources, environmental pollution, and overpopulation. Those problems threaten your personal success and they cannot be solved with the same way of thinking that has created them. Therefore, Lao Zi's Dao De Jing is more relevant than ever. His way of dynamic thinking fosters solutions that reach peacefully across the fault-lines created by race, religion, and ideology. This book is based on (Schade, Lao Zi's Dao De Jing Demystified, 2017).

Ancient Theory ... Physics [4]

Two-and-halve thousand years ago, Lao Zi wrote Dao De Jing. His demystified book shows that he was the first to describe scientific concepts including: gravity, antimatter, nothingness, fluctuation, and a zero-sum creation theory. His creation Theory of Fluctuating Nothingness holds that Nothingness was divided into the mirror universes of Matter and Antimatter. Their fluctuation around Nothingness creates a temporal buffer that prevents their mutual annihilation and conceals Antimatter from perception. The constancy of Nothingness underlies the cosmic balance between matter and antimatter. That balance is maintained by the force Qi, which comprises the gravitational, electro-magnetic, and nuclear forces. Movements such as reactions, entropy, and chaos are manifestations of that balancing process. Lao Zi's ancient theory challenges the history, purpose, methodology, and philosophical premises of modern physics. The purpose of Dao or physics is obtaining knowledge about nature. On the other hand, the purpose of De or psychology is obtaining wisdom in order to apply that knowledge productively. Lao Zi's theories are relative to our era, because they foster crucial research in several scientific fields that could help the next generation to face manmade extinction problems.

Ancient Theory ... Psychology [11]

About two-and-halve thousand years ago, Lao Zi wrote Dao De Jing, which means: A Classic about the Physics of Psychology. His aim is to maximize success, which he defined as to obtain what you seek and escape what you suffer. Unfortunately, scholars have mystified his book by explaining his scientific theories in supernatural terminology. Manmade extinction problems, such as nuclear war and climate change, show that humanity suffers from systemic cognitive failure. Those problems cannot be solved with the same way of thinking that has created them. Humanity needs a valid and reliable theory for problem solving. Lao Zi's Theory of Fluctuating Nothingness provides a rationale for modern physics. His theory holds that balance is the cosmic principle, while the force Qi maintains and restores that balance. Qi comprises the gravitational, electro-magnetic, and nuclear forces. People maximize their success by aligning with the unstoppable Qi. Therefore, physics is the only valid and reliable basis for psychology. The aim of this study is to evaluate Lao Zi's Cognitive Criteria for Problem-solving. Those criteria include: focus, balance, efficiency, and proactivity.

The Cognitive Revolution [12]

For many millennia, humanity has lived in a relatively static reality. However, during the last few centuries, education has fostered the science and technology that has turned that static reality into the modern hyperdynamic one. Unfortunately, the cognitive adjustment to that environmental dynamism lags behind. As a result, people have become static thinkers in a hyperdynamic reality. That contradiction has created manmade extinction problems such as nuclear war and climate change. Such threats of self-destruction are scientific evidence that humanity suffers from systemic cognitive failure. Despite the advantages of the educational system, it is complicit in those threats. Science and technology might not be the answer. Although computers are fast, they are unlikely to solve those complex extinction problems, because they are simplified replicas of the human mind. Instead, the educational system should adopt a way of thinking that fits the hyperdynamic reality. Based on ideas of Lao Zi, Aristotle, and Hegel; the Cognitive Accelerator is introduced in order to foster the cognitive revolution from Static to Dynamic Thinking. Humanity needs a revolution, because it is rapidly running out of time.

Education Kills Humanity [13]

The aim of this study is to evaluate the educational system with nemonik thinking (Schade, Think Smarter with Nemonik Thinking, 2016). The system conditions students with certificates to maximize their probability of winning the educational competition. The winners are rewarded with advantageous positions in society, while the losers are doomed to serve the winners. Therefore, conventional thinking is conflict oriented, which fosters aggression, control, effort, and force. The conditioned compulsion to win arguments inhibits also the truth and, therefore, it corrupts conventional thinking. As a result, the educational system produces incompetent leaders and rebellious followers. That counterproductive combination fosters manmade problems such as climate change, continuous warfare, dwindling resources, environmental pollution, and overpopulation. Those problems cannot be solved with the same way of conventional thinking that has created them. In contrast, nemonik thinking aims for success, rather than winning. Success is to obtain what you seek and to escape what you suffer. Therefore, nemonik thinking is goal oriented, which fosters freedom, alignment, compassion, allies, and win-win strategies. You might be the best thinker in the world, but only nemonik thinking could make you the smartest thinker you can be. This book contains extracts from (Schade, Think Smarter with Nemonik Thinking, 2016).

Maximum Success with Nemonik Thinking [2]

Nemonik Thinking will maximize your success with a minimum of effort and resources. Success is to obtain what you seek and escape what you suffer. Manmade extinction problems, such as nuclear war and climate change, are evidence that humanity's way of Conventional Thinking is failing. Conventional Thinking is a poorly understood, corrupted, and outdated set of cognitive tools that maintains static thinking in a hyperdynamic reality. Unfortunately, that is what they taught you at school. Hence, you will need this handbook, because that will make you the best thinker you can be. Nemonik thinking is for the brain what Windows is for the computer. It is a unique cognitive operating system that comprises dynamic thinking and mind management. Dynamic thinking maximizes your external success with an exhaustive checklist of 21 keywords that activate a set of efficient problem-solving tools. On the other hand, mind management maximizes your internal success with concentrated-relaxation and mantras. Nemonik Thinking is as objective as logic and algebra, but a lot easier to learn and apply. It offers the only realistic protection for your life, family, and assets within our hyperdynamic reality. Nemonik Thinking sounds like magic, because it is.

Survival [3]

(eBook: Extinction SOS)

Your life, family, and assets are in great danger. Humans are the apex predators on this planet. Despite our morality and knowledge, we kill each other by the millions, drive other species towards extinction, and destroy even our own habitat. Asking people to become peaceful is like asking tigers to become vegetarians.

Our technology has changed the static reality of the past into today's hyperdynamic one. However, manmade extinction problems, such as nuclear war and climate change, show that the educational way of thinking remained static. That has to improve, because those self-destructive problems cannot be solved with the failing way of thinking that has created them.

Humanity is rapidly running out of time, because groupthink and cognitive dissonance maintain the threat. Therefore, the psychologist Dr Auke Schade has launched Nemonik Thinking. That unique mindware provides a competitive advantage that will turn weaknesses into strengths and threats into opportunities. It will maximize success by making people the best thinkers they can be. Success is to obtain what we seek and escape what we suffer.

Knowledge [9]

(eBook Science)

Knowledge is a valid and reliable description of reality. On the other hand, wisdom is the productive application of knowledge. Lao Zi's Dao De Jing means A Classic about the Physics of Psychology. He proposed that knowledge should be based on the simple principle of balance. In contrast, Aristotle developed logic, which is described in the Organon meaning The Instrument. Logic requires factual details in order to create new knowledge. Unfortunately, educational thinking propagates static thinking in our hyperdynamic reality. Science is forced to deal with an infinite number of details that fragments science. Technology applies knowledge without adequate wisdom. Those failures fuel the triangle of doom. Education fosters science, science fosters technology, and technology creates manmade extinction problems such as nuclear war and climate change. Those problems show that humanity suffers from systemic cognitive failure. That failure is maintained by institutionalization, groupthink, and cognitive dissonance. Our problems cannot be solved with just more of the same education, science, and technology. Humanity needs a new paradigm of thinking that creates the next generation of thinkers. Therefore, Nemonik Thinking synthesizes Lao Zi's and Aristotle's ideas about thinking, knowledge, and wisdom.

Simplification [13]

Synonyms are words with a similar meaning that prevent boring repetitions. They are useful for writing books and making speeches. For example, 'advancing' could be replaced subsequently with forward, proceeding, progressing, evolving, etc. Nevertheless, the huge number of synonyms creates a cognitive noise that hinders problem-solving. Imagine that the 120,000 words of the Oxford Dictionary were printed in random order. How long would it take you to find a particular word in that chaos? Fortunately, the words are sorted in alphabetical order. Therefore, you have only to search less than 4% of the words. As a result, it will take only a few seconds to locate any specific word in that dictionary. However, the brain is infinitely more complex than any dictionary. It is a huge organic computer with billions of neurons each one interconnected with multiple synapses. Unfortunately, the conscious has no natural system that controls the storing, recalling, and processing of mental information. Apparently, it just happens. In order to reduce the mental noise, Nemonik Thinking simplifies the thousands of synonyms to a checklist of 21 memorized prompts called nemoniks. Those nemoniks are exhaustive, because they cover every possible aspect of thinking including Lao Zi's dynamic balance, mind, reality, and their interaction. Recalling a nemonik activates guided-association between that nemonik and relative problem-solving tools.

Add Your own Proverbs

Made in the USA
Las Vegas, NV
03 November 2026

57421650R00169